MW00892321

RENAL DIET COOKBOOK FOR BEGINNER

Unlock the Power of Kidney Health. 1800 Days of Low Potassium, Sodium, and Phosphorus Delights. A Life-Changing 8-Week Meal Plan. Healthy Kidney, Flavorful Healing

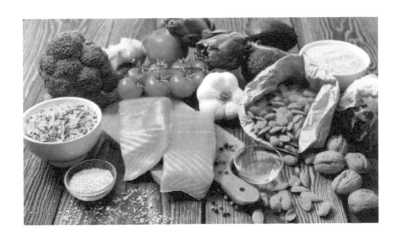

Sophia Mitchell

Copryright © 2023 by Sophia Mitchell. All rights reserved

RENAL DIET DIET COOKBOOK FOR BEGINNERS

ISBN: 9798859020539

All right Reserved

FREE BONUS

The Habits that damage your Kidneys

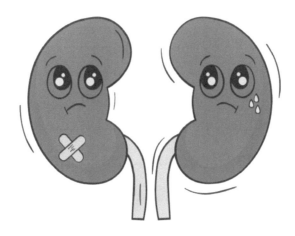

Mastering the Right Mindset for your Renal Diet Journey

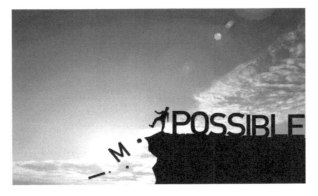

https://free-bonus.biz

Table of Contents

Introduction

Introduction to Kidney Health and The Kidney Diet

For individuals facing impaired kidney function, maintaining a specific diet is essential to combat the accumulation of waste in their bloodstream. The waste substances stem from the consumption of food and beverages. When kidney function is compromised, the kidneys struggle to efficiently filter and eliminate this waste. Unfortunately, the presence of waste in the blood can negatively impact the patient's electrolyte levels. However, there is a glimmer of hope. By adhering to a renal diet, individuals have the potential to boost kidney function and impede the progression towards complete kidney failure.

A renal diet is distinguished by its low levels of sodium, phosphorus, and protein. In addition to this, it highlights the significance of taking protein of a high grade whilst usually reducing the amount of fluid consumed. There is a possibility that certain patients will furthermore require a reduction in the amount of potassium and calcium they consume. It is essential for patients to work together with a renal dietitian in order to design a personalized diet that meets their particular needs. This is due to the fact that the human body is distinct for every individual.

The Kidneys and Their Role in Overall Health

The kidneys are responsible for filtering the blood and removing waste products before sending the blood that has been cleansed back to the rest of the body. Each min, the renal arteries allow roughly a liter of blood, that is one-fifth of the amount of blood that flows by the heart, to make it to the kidneys. This blood is supplied by the heart. After being purified, the blood travels via the renal veins back to the rest of the body.

Nephrons are the name given to the roughly one million tiny units that make up every kidney. A glomerulus, often known as a microscopic filter, and a tubule are the two components that make up each nephron. Nephrons act as filters, removing fluid and waste items from the blood as it travels across the kidney. After that, the majority of the fluid goes back into the blood, and the waste products are gathered in any extra fluid that is passed out of the body as urine.

Urine reaches the bladder after passing via a tube known as the ureter and before reaching the kidneys. Urine is then released from the body via the urethra, which is located at the base of the bladder. Based on parameters like body size, level of hydration, temperature, and level of physical activity, the kidneys normally generate between one and two liters of pee on a daily basis.

When the kidneys are healthy, their functional capability can be greatly increased. When both kidneys are healthy, each kidney is responsible for carrying out fifty percent of the typical renal function. If one kidney is removed, the other kidney may make up by growing larger and performing as much as seventy-five percent of the usual kidney function. This is the same amount of work that would be done by one and a half kidneys if they were both healthy and operating regularly.

Common Kidney Problems and The Importance of Diet in Managing Kidney Health

Kidney problems are a common health issue affecting millions of people worldwide. The kidneys are responsible for a number of important bodily functions, including the removal of waste products and extra fluid from the circulation, the regulation of blood pressure, and the maintenance of electrolyte balance. When the kidneys are not functioning properly, various health conditions can arise.

One of the most prevalent kidney problems is chronic kidney disease (CKD), which occurs when the kidneys slowly lose their aptitude to function over time. CKD is often caused by conditions like diabetes, high blood pressure, and certain genetic disorders. Another common issue is kidney stones, which are hard deposits that form in the kidneys and can cause severe pain and discomfort. Urinary tract infections (UTIs) can also affect the kidneys if left untreated, leading to kidney infection or inflammation.

Diet plays a crucial role in managing kidney health. For individuals with kidney problems, it is essential to follow a kidney-friendly diet that helps maintain optimal kidney function and prevents further damage. A kidney-friendly diet typically involves controlling the intake of certain nutrients such as sodium, potassium, and phosphorus.

Reducing sodium intake is important to manage blood pressure and fluid balance. This involves limiting processed and packaged foods, which are often high in sodium, and opting for fresh, homemade meals with minimal salt. Potassium levels should also be regulated, as excessive potassium can be harmful to the kidneys. Foods like bananas, oranges, tomatoes, and potatoes, which are high in potassium, should be consumed in moderation.

Phosphorus, found in many foods like dairy products, nuts, and carbonated drinks, should also be monitored. High phosphorus levels can contribute to mineral and bone disorders in kidney patients. It is advisable to limit phosphorus-rich foods and opt for lower-phosphorus alternatives.

Maintaining a healthy weight, staying hydrated, and limiting alcohol consumption are important for kidney health. It is crucial for individuals with kidney problems to work closely with healthcare professionals and registered dietitians to develop personalized diet plans that suit their specific needs and medical conditions.

What Is A Renal Diet and How It Works

A renal diet assists in maintaining proper kidney function for individuals suffering from kidney disease. Positioned below the ribcage on either side of the spine, the kidneys, resembling beans in shape, carry out vital tasks, including filtering the blood, eliminating waste through urine, and regulating fluid balance in the body. When kidney disease is present, the kidneys are unable to filter the blood effectively, resulting in an accumulation of excessive amounts of sodium, potassium, phosphorus, and protein byproducts in the bloodstream. This accumulation can exacerbate kidney damage and lead to fluid retention.

A renal diet involves reducing the intake of protein, sodium, potassium, and phosphorus. By adhering to this diet, the workload on the kidneys is reduced, promoting their health. Additionally, it aids in managing fluid levels in the body, preventing excessive fluid retention.

The degree of kidney damage determines the maximum amounts of protein, salt, potassium, and phosphorus that can be consumed on a daily basis. In the event that your kidney disease has progressed to an extensive stage, your physician should advise you with the essential limits and constraints.

Key Principles of The Renal Diet

The renal diet, also known as the kidney diet, is specifically designed to manage kidney health and prevent further complications in individuals with kidney problems, such as chronic kidney disease (CKD). The key principles of the renal diet involve limiting the intake of sodium, potassium, phosphorus, and protein. Here's a brief overview of these principles:

1. Sodium: Sodium restriction is crucial in managing blood pressure and fluid balance. An excessive consumption of salt could cause fluid retention as well as a rise in blood pressure, which can put additional strain on the kidneys. The renal diet emphasizes avoiding or reducing processed and packaged foods, as they often contain high amounts of sodium. Instead, choosing fresh and homemade meals with minimal salt is recommended. Using herbs, spices, and other flavorings can help enhance the taste of low-sodium dishes.

2. Potassium: Potassium levels need to be regulated in the renal diet, as high potassium levels can be harmful to the kidneys and lead to various complications. Foods rich in potassium, such as bananas, oranges, tomatoes, potatoes, and avocados, should be consumed in moderation. Cooking methods like boiling or soaking vegetables in water can help reduce their potassium content. It's important to work with a healthcare professional or dietitian to determine an appropriate potassium intake based on individual needs.

3. Phosphorus: High phosphorus levels can contribute to mineral and bone disorders in individuals with kidney problems. The renal diet involves limiting phosphorus-rich foods such as dairy products, nuts, seeds, carbonated drinks, and processed foods. Instead, choosing lower-phosphorus alternatives like lean meats, poultry, fish, and fresh fruits and vegetables is recommended. Phosphorus binders may also be prescribed by healthcare professionals to help control phosphorus levels.

4. Protein: Protein restriction is often advised in the renal diet, particularly in advanced stages of kidney disease. High-protein diets can increase the workload on the kidneys and result in the accumulation of waste products. However, protein needs may vary based on the stage of kidney disease and individual factors. Healthcare professionals or dietitians can determine the appropriate protein intake and recommend sources of high-quality protein, like lean meats, poultry, fish, eggs, and dairy products.

List of Healthy Foods and Nutrients for Kidney Health

Protein options: Protein is crucial for maintaining kidney health, but it's important not to consume excessive amounts if your kidneys have difficulty eliminating waste. Typically, it is safe to have a small portion of protein with each meal. A dietitian can assess whether you should increase or decrease your protein intake.

Here are some recommended protein choices:

- Skinless chicken or turkey.
- Fish or seafood.
- Lean beef such as sirloin or tenderloin.
- Eggs.
- Tofu and beans, such as kidney beans or lentils. Note that these options have higher levels of potassium and phosphorus, so portion sizes may need to be limited.

Fruit and vegetable choices: Many fruits and vegetables contain high levels of potassium, and you may need to either avoid them or consume smaller portions. Consulting with a renal dietitian is best, as they can guide you on which fruits and vegetables to eat and in what quantities. Some delicious lower-potassium fruit and vegetable options include:

- Apples
- Blackberries
- Blueberries
- Cherries
- Grapes
- Pineapple
- Strawberries
- Tangerines
- Green beans
- Cabbage
- Cucumbers
- Eggplant
- Kale
- Lettuce
- Sweet peppers
- Zucchini

Options for grains and starches: While whole grains are a good source of fiber, vitamins, and minerals, numerous kinds of these grains have a high potassium content. As a result, you might have to cut back on the amount you eat and the number of times you consume the food. The following are some choices that are healthier and lower in potassium:

- Barley
- Buckwheat
- Bulgur
- Wild rice
- Unsalted popcorn

White bread, pasta, or rice have lower potassium levels compared to their whole-grain counterparts. To determine if these options are more suitable for you, consult with your dietitian.

Foods That Should Be Limited or Avoided in A Renal Diet

Many snack foods and convenience foods that come in packages or cans have a high sodium content. The same applies to processed meats, seasoned meats, and pickled vegetables. It is advisable to read the nutrition facts label and choose foods that contain less than 240 mg of sodium per serving. Here are some high-sodium foods that you should avoid or consume in limited quantities:

- Chips, crackers, pretzels, and salted popcorn.
- Canned soups or stews.
- Pickles, olives, pickled vegetables, or relishes.
- Deli meats and cheeses (unless labeled as "low sodium"), hot dogs, sausages, and bacon.
- Packaged meals such as frozen dinners or mac and cheese.
- Packaged, seasoned rice or noodles.
- Frozen, seasoned meats or fish like chicken strips or fish sticks.

In addition, it is advisable to limit the consumption of high-potassium foods, such as:

- Apricots.
- Bananas.
- Cantaloupe.
- Dried fruits.
- Honeydew.
- Kiwi.
- Nectarines.
- Oranges.
- Broccoli.
- Carrots.
- Parsnips.
- Potatoes (white and sweet).
- Spinach.
- Tomatoes (including tomato sauce or juice).

- Winter squash.

- Nuts and nut butters.

- Seeds like sunflower or pumpkin seeds.

- Chocolate.

- Molasses.

- Granola and bran cereals.

- Salt substitutes that contain potassium.

Lastly, on a renal diet, it may be necessary to limit the portions of high-phosphorus foods, such as:

- Dairy products like milk, yogurt, cheese, or ice cream.

- Dried beans like kidney, black, or pinto beans.

- Mushrooms.

- Cocoa.

- Beer.

- Dark soft drinks like colas or root beers.

It's worth noting that oat milk and milk substitutes have gained popularity, but depending on the brand, oat milk can contain up to 20% phosphorus.

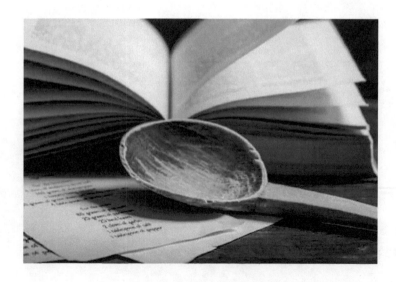

Breakfast Recipes

Spinach and Feta Egg Muffins

Degree of Difficulty: ★★★☆☆

Preparation time: ten mins

Cooking time: twenty-five mins

Servings: 3

Ingredients:

- 6 eggs
- half teacup chopped spinach
- quarter teacup crumbled feta cheese
- quarter teacup diced tomatoes
- Salt and pepper as required
- Olive oil (for greasing the muffin tin)

Directions:

1. Warm up the oven to 350°F.
2. Oil a muffin tin with olive oil.
3. Inside your container, beat the eggs and flavour with salt and pepper.
4. Stir in the chopped spinach, crumbled feta cheese, and diced tomatoes.
5. Transfer the egg mixture into the greased muffin tin, filling each cup about 2/3 full.
6. Bake for around twenty to twenty-five mins or till the egg muffins are cooked and lightly golden.
7. Take out from the oven and let them cool for a couple of mins prior to removing from the muffin tin.
8. Serve warm or at room temp.

Per serving: Calories: 140kcal; Fat: 10g; Carbs: 2g; Protein: 11g; Sugar: 1g; Sodium: 150mg; Potassium: 170mg; Phosphorus: 180mg

Oatmeal with Fresh Berries

Degree of Difficulty: ★☆☆☆☆

Preparation time: five mins

Cooking time: ten mins

Servings: one

Ingredients:

- half teacup rolled oats
- one teacup water
- quarter teacup fresh berries (e.g., strawberries, blueberries, raspberries)
- 1 tablespoon chopped walnuts
- Cinnamon (optional)

Directions:

1. In your small pot, bring water to a boil.
2. Include the rolled oats then decrease the temp. to low.
3. Cook the oats for 5 mins, mixing irregularly.
4. Take out from temp. and let it relax for a min.

5. Top with fresh berries, chopped walnuts, and a sprinkle of cinnamon if desired.

6. Serve warm.

Per serving: Calories: 230kcal; Fat: 8g; Carbs: 34g; Protein: 7g; Sugar: 3g; Sodium: 0mg; Potassium: 120mg; Phosphorus: 160mg

Cottage Cheese with Fresh Fruit

Degree of Difficulty: ★★★★★

Preparation time: five mins

Cooking time: zero mins

Servings: 1

Ingredients:

- half teacup low-fat cottage cheese
- quarter teacup diced fresh fruit (e.g., melon, pineapple, grapes)
- 1 tablespoon chopped walnuts
- 1 teaspoon honey (optional)

Directions:

1. Inside a container, place the cottage cheese.

2. Top with diced fresh fruit and chopped walnuts.

3. Spray with honey if desired.

4. Serve chilled.

Per serving: Calories: 160kcal; Fat: 6g; Carbs: 14g; Protein: 15g; Sugar: 11g; Sodium: 280mg; Potassium: 180mg; Phosphorus: 180mg

Egg and Vegetable Muffins

Degree of Difficulty: ★★★☆☆

Preparation time: fifteen mins

Cooking time: twenty mins

Servings: six

Ingredients:

- 6 eggs
- quarter teacup cubed bell peppers
- quarter teacup cubed zucchini
- quarter teacup cubed onions
- quarter teacup cubed tomatoes
- Salt and pepper as required
- Olive oil (for greasing the muffin tin)

Directions:

1. Warm up the oven to 350°F.

2. Oil a muffin tin with olive oil.

3. Inside your container, beat the eggs and flavour with salt and pepper.

4. Stir in the cubed bell peppers, zucchini, onions, and tomatoes.

5. Pour the egg & vegetable mixture into the greased muffin tin, filling all cup about 2/3 full.

6. Bake for around fifteen-twenty mins or 'til the egg muffins are cooked and lightly golden.

7. Take out from the oven and allow them to cool for a couple of mins prior to removing from the muffin tin.

8. Serve warm or at room temp.

Per serving: Calories: 110kcal; Fat: 7g; Carbs: 4gm; Protein: 8g; Sugar: 2g; Sodium: 90mg; Potassium: 160mg; Phosphorus: 110mg

Fruit Salad with Mint

Degree of Difficulty: ★☆☆☆☆

Preparation time: ten mins

Cooking time: zero mins

Servings: 2

Ingredients:

- half teacup cubed melon
- half teacup cubed pineapple
- half teacup cubed grapes
- quarter teacup fresh mint leaves, chopped
- 1 teaspoon lime juice

Directions:

1. Inside a container, blend the cubed melon, pineapple, grapes, and chopped mint leaves.
2. Spray with lime juice and throw gently to blend.
3. Serve cooled.

Per serving: Calories: 80kcal; Fat: 0g; Carbs: 20g; Protein: 1gm; Sugar: 17g; Sodium: 0mg; Potassium: 240mg; Phosphorus: 30mg

Sweet Potato Hash Browns

Degree of Difficulty: ★★★☆☆

Preparation time: fifteen mins

Cooking time: twenty mins

Servings: two

Ingredients:

- 1 medium sweet potato, grated
- quarter teacup cubed onions
- quarter teacup cubed bell peppers
- Salt and pepper as required
- Olive oil (for cooking)

Directions:

1. Inside a big container, blend the grated sweet potato, cubed onions, cubed bell peppers, salt, and pepper.
2. Warm a non-stick griddle in a middling temp. then include a small amount of olive oil.
3. Get a handful of the sweet potato mixture then squeeze out any excess liquid.
4. Place the squeezed mixture into the griddle and level it with a spatula to form a hash brown.
5. Cook for around five to seven mins on all sides till the hash brown is golden and crispy.
6. Replicate with the remaining sweet potato mixture.
7. Serve hot.

Per serving: Calories: 180kcal; Fat: 6g; Carbs: 30g; Protein: 3gm; Sugar: 9g; Sodium: 70mg; Potassium: 330mg; Phosphorus: 70mg

Yogurt Parfait

Degree of Difficulty: ★★★★★

Preparation time: five mins

Cooking time: zero mins

Servings: 1

Ingredients:

- half teacup low-fat plain yogurt
- quarter teacup fresh berries (e.g., strawberries, blueberries, raspberries)
- 1 tablespoon chopped almonds
- 1 tablespoon ground flaxseed (optional)

Directions:

1. In your glass or container, layer half of the yogurt.
2. Include half of the fresh berries on top of the yogurt.
3. Include the remaining yogurt and top with the remaining fresh berries.
4. Sprinkle with chopped almonds and ground flaxseed (if using).
5. Serve cooled.

Per serving: Calories: 180kcal; Fat: 7g; Carbs: 19g; Protein: 11gm; Sugar: 8g; Sodium: 80mg; Potassium: 280mg; Phosphorus: 180mg

Shrimp Bruschetta

Degree of Difficulty: ★★☆☆☆

Preparation time: fifteen mins

Cooking time: ten mins

Servings: four

Ingredients:

- 13 oz. shrimps, peeled
- 1 tablespoon tomato sauce
- ½ teaspoon Splenda
- ¼ teaspoon garlic powder
- 1 teaspoon fresh parsley, chopped
- ½ teaspoon olive oil
- 1 teaspoon lemon juice
- 4 whole-grain bread slices
- one teacup water, for cooking

Directions:

1. In the saucepan, pour water and raise it to boil.
2. Include shrimps and boil them over the high heat for five mins.
3. After this, drain shrimps and chill them to the room temperature.
4. Mix up together shrimps with Splenda, garlic powder, tomato sauce, and fresh parsley.
5. Include lemon juice and stir gently.
6. Warm up the oven to 360 deg. F.
7. Coat the slice of bread with olive oil and bake for 3 minutes.
8. Then place the shrimp mixture on the bread. Bruschetta is cooked.

Per serving: Calories: 199kcal; Fat: 3.7g; Carbs: 15.3g; Protein: 24.1g; Sugar: 6g; Sodium: 121mg; Potassium: 227mg; Phosphorus: 316mg

Vegetable and Egg Wrap

Degree of Difficulty: ★★☆☆☆

Preparation time: ten mins

Cooking time: ten mins

Servings: one

Ingredients:

- one whole wheat tortilla
- 2 eggs, scrambled
- quarter teacup cubed bell peppers
- quarter teacup cubed onions
- quarter teacup cubed tomatoes
- Salt and pepper as required
- Olive oil (for cooking)

Directions:

1. Inside a non-stick griddle, heat a small amount of olive oil across middling temp.
2. Include the cubed bell peppers, onions, and tomatoes. Sauté till they are tender.
3. Inside a container, scramble the eggs and flavour with salt and pepper.
4. Push the cooked vegetables to one side of the griddle then place the beaten eggs to the other side.
5. Cook the eggs, mixing irregularly 'til they are fully cooked.
6. Warm the whole wheat tortilla in a separate pan or microwave.
7. Spread the scrambled eggs and sautéed vegetables onto the tortilla.
8. Roll up the tortilla into a wrap.
9. Serve warm.

Per serving: Calories: 320kcal; Fat: 14g; Carbs: 32g; Protein: 18g; Sugar: 8g; Sodium: 280mg; Potassium: 300mg; Phosphorus: 200mg

Scrambled Eggs with Vegetables

Degree of Difficulty: ★★☆☆☆

Preparation time: five mins

Cooking time: ten mins

Servings: one

Ingredients:

- 2 eggs
- quarter teacup cubed bell peppers
- quarter teacup cubed onions
- quarter teacup cubed zucchini
- Salt-free seasoning blend
- Olive oil (for cooking)

Directions:

1. Inside a non-stick pot, heat a small amount of olive oil across middling temp.
2. Include the cubed vegetables then cook till they are soft.
3. Inside your container, whisk the eggs and include them to the pan with the cooked vegetables.
4. Stir gently till the eggs are cooked to your anticipated consistency.
5. Season with salt-free seasoning blend.
6. Serve hot.

Per serving: Calories: 210kcal; Fat: 14g; Carbs: 9g; Protein: 13g; Sugar: 5gm; Sodium: 60mg; Potassium: 280mg; Phosphorus: 180mg

Vegetable Frittata

Degree of Difficulty: ★★★☆☆

Preparation time: ten mins

Cooking time: twenty-five mins

Servings: two

Ingredients:

- 4 eggs
- quarter teacup cubed tomatoes
- quarter teacup cubed bell peppers
- quarter teacup cubed onions
- quarter teacup cubed mushrooms
- two tbsps chopped fresh parsley
- Salt and pepper as required
- Olive oil (for cooking)

Directions:

1. Warm up the oven to 350°F.
2. Inside your container, whisk the eggs and flavour with salt and pepper.
3. Inside a non-stick griddle, warm a small amount of olive oil across middling temp.
4. Include the cubed vegetables then cook till they are soft.
5. Pour the whisked eggs over the cooked vegetables in the griddle.
6. Cook for 2-3 minutes 'til the edges start to set.

7. Transmit the griddle to the warmed up oven then bake for around twenty mins or till the eggs are fully set.
8. Spray with fresh parsley prior to serving.

Per serving: Calories: 230kcal; Fat: 15g; Carbs: 10g; Protein: 15g; Sugar: 5g; Sodium: 180mg; Potassium: 280mg; Phosphorus: 220mg

Quinoa Breakfast Bowl

Degree of Difficulty: ★★★☆☆

Preparation time: ten mins

Cooking time: fifteen mins

Servings: one

Ingredients:

- quarter teacup quinoa
- half teacup water
- quarter teacup cubed apples
- one tbsp chopped almonds
- one tbsp dried cranberries
- quarter tsp cinnamon
- quarter teacup low-fat milk or an almond milk

Directions:

1. Wash the quinoa below cold water.
2. Inside a small pot, raise the water to a boil.
3. Place the quinoa to the boiling water, decrease temp. to low, and cover.
4. Simmer for around fifteen mins or till the quinoa is cooked and the water is immersed.

5. Inside a container, blend the cooked quinoa, cubed apples, chopped almonds, dried cranberries, cinnamon, and milk.

6. Stir well to blend.

7. Serve warm.

Per serving: Calories: 220kcal; Fat: 7g; Carbs: 34g; Protein: 7g; Sugar: 10g; Sodium: 10mg; Potassium: 200mg; Phosphorus: 160mg

Cinnamon Apple Pancakes

Degree of Difficulty: ★★☆☆☆

Preparation time: fifteen mins

Cooking time: ten mins

Servings: 2

Ingredients:

- half teacup whole wheat flour
- half tsp baking powder
- half tsp ground cinnamon
- quarter tsp salt
- half teacup low-fat milk or an almond milk
- one tbsp unsweetened applesauce
- half tsp vanilla extract
- one small apple, skinned and grated
- Olive oil (for cooking)

Directions:

1. Inside your container, whisk collectively the whole wheat flour, baking powder, ground cinnamon, and salt.

2. Inside a separate container, blend the low-fat milk, applesauce & vanilla extract.

3. Bring the wet components into the dry components and stir till just blended.

4. Fold in the grated apple.

5. Heat a non-stick griddle in a middling temp. then include a small quantity of olive oil.

6. Place a quarter teacup of the batter into the griddle to form all pancakes.

7. Cook 'til bubbles form on the surface, afterwards flip then cook for an extra min or till golden brown.

8. Replicate with the rest of the batter.

9. Serve the pancakes warm.

Per serving: Calories: 190kcal; Fat: 2g; Carbs: 38g; Protein: 6g; Sugar: 9g; Sodium: 200mg; Potassium: 320mg; Phosphorus: 180mg

Whole Wheat Toast with Avocado

Degree of Difficulty: ★☆☆☆☆

Preparation time: five mins

Cooking time: zero mins

Servings: one

Ingredients:

- one slice of whole wheat bread
- 1/4 avocado, mashed
- half tsp lemon juice
- Salt and pepper as required

Directions:

1. Toast the whole wheat bread till golden.

2. Inside your container, mash the avocado with lemon juice, salt & pepper.

3. Spread the mashed avocado on top of the toasted bread.

4. Serve immediately.

Per serving: Calories: 160kcal; Fat: 9g; Carbs: 18g; Protein: 4g; Sugar: 1g; Sodium: 100mg; Potassium: 240mg; Phosphorus: 100mg

Easy Turnip Puree

Degree of Difficulty: ★★☆☆☆

Preparation time: ten mins

Cooking time: twelve mins

Servings: four

Ingredients:

- one and half lbs. turnips, skinned and chopped
- 1 tsp. dill
- 3 bacon slices, cooked and chopped
- 2 tbsp. fresh chives, chopped

Directions:

1. Include turnip into the boiling water and cook for twelve mins. Drain thoroughly then place inside a mixing container.

2. Include dill and process till even.

3. Transfer turnip puree into the container and top with bacon and chives.

4. Serve and relish.

Per serving: Calories: 127kcal; Fat: 6gm; Carbs: 11.6g; Protein: 6.8g; Sugar: 7g; Sodium: 86mg; Potassium: 127mg; Phosphorus: 110mg

Blueberry Chia Pudding

Degree of Difficulty: ★★☆☆☆

Preparation time: ten mins

Cooking time: zero mins

Servings: two

Ingredients:

- quarter teacup chia seeds
- one teacup low-fat milk or almond milk
- one tbsp honey or maple syrup
- half tsp vanilla extract
- half teacup fresh blueberries

Directions:

1. In a blender, blend the fresh blueberries till even.

2. Inside your container, blend the chia seeds, milk, honey or maple syrup, and vanilla extract.

3. Whisk well till everything is well blended.

4. Include the blended blueberries to the chia mixture and stir till evenly distributed.

5. Cover the container and put in the fridge for almost four hrs or overnight, letting the chia seeds to absorb the liquid and thicken.

6. Stir the chia pudding prior to serving to distribute the seeds and blueberries.

7. Serve cooled.

Per serving: Calories: 160kcal; Fat: 6g; Carbs: 21g; Protein: 5g; Sugar: 11g; Sodium: 50mg; Potassium: 220mg; Phosphorus: 130mg

Veggie Breakfast Burrito

Degree of Difficulty: ★★★☆☆

Preparation time: fifteen mins

Cooking time: ten mins

Servings: one

Ingredients:

- one complete wheat tortilla
- 2 eggs, scrambled
- quarter teacup cubed bell peppers
- quarter teacup cubed onions
- quarter teacup cubed tomatoes
- quarter teacup cubed zucchini
- Salt and pepper as required
- Olive oil (for cooking)

Directions:

1. Inside a non-stick griddle, heat a small quantity of olive oil across middling temp.

2. Include the cubed bell peppers, onions, tomatoes, and zucchini. Sauté till they are soft.

3. Inside a container, scramble the eggs and flavour with salt and pepper.

4. After the vegetables have finished cooking, move them to one end of the griddle, and then transfer the whisked eggs to the opposite end.

5. Cook the eggs, mixing irregularly 'til they are fully cooked.

6. Warm the whole wheat tortilla in a separate pan or microwave.

7. Spread the scrambled eggs and sautéed vegetables onto the tortilla.

8. Roll up the tortilla into a burrito.

9. Serve warm.

Per serving: Calories: 320kcal; Fat: 14g; Carbs: 32g; Protein: 18g; Sugar: 8g; Sodium: 280mg; Potassium: 300mg; Phosphorus: 200mg

Berry Smoothie

Degree of Difficulty: ★☆☆☆☆

Preparation time: five mins

Cooking time: zero mins

Servings: 1

Ingredients:

- half teacup frozen mixed berries (e.g., strawberries, blueberries, raspberries)
- half teacup low-fat milk or an almond milk
- quarter teacup low-fat Greek yogurt
- one tbsp ground flaxseed

Directions:

1. Inside a mixer, blend the frozen mixed berries, milk, Greek yogurt, and ground flaxseed.

2. Blend till even and creamy.

3. If anticipated, place more milk for a thinner consistency.

4. Pour into a glass and serve instantly.

Per serving: Calories: 160kcal; Fat: 6g; Carbs: 17g; Protein: 10g; Sugar: 10g; Sodium: 90mg; Potassium: 260mg; Phosphorus: 170mg

Greek Yogurt with Honey and Nuts

Degree of Difficulty: ★★★★☆

Preparation time: five mins

Cooking time: zero mins

Servings: 1

Ingredients:

- half teacup low-fat Greek yogurt
- one tbsp chopped almonds
- one tbsp severed walnuts- one tsp honey

Directions:

1. Inside a container, place the Greek yogurt.
2. Top with severed almonds and walnuts.
3. Spray with honey.
4. Serve cooled.

Per serving: Calories: 180kcal; Fat: 10g; Carbs: 10g; Protein: 15g; Sugar: 8g; Sodium: 70mg; Potassium: 200mg; Phosphorus: 180mg

Ham and Cheese Omelet

Degree of Difficulty: ★★☆☆☆

Preparation time: ten mins

Cooking time: ten mins

Servings: one

Ingredients:

- 2 eggs
- quarter teacup cubed ham
- quarter teacup shredded low-sodium cheese (e.g., cheddar, Swiss)
- Salt and pepper as required
- Olive oil (for cooking)

Directions:

1. Inside your container, whisk the eggs then flavour with salt and pepper.
2. Warm a non-stick griddle in a middling temp. then include a small quantity of olive oil.
3. Include the cubed ham to the griddle and cook for a couple of mins till it starts to brown.
4. Pour the whisked eggs over the ham in the griddle.
5. Cook for a couple of mins till the edges start to set.
6. Spray the shredded cheese over the eggs.
7. Gently lift the edges of the omelet then tilt the griddle to let the uncooked eggs to flow to the edges.
8. Cook till the eggs are fully set and the cheese is dissolved.
9. Wrap the omelet in half and transfer to a plate.
10. Serve hot.

Per serving: Calories: 280kcal; Fat: 20g; Carbs: 3g; Protein: 21g; Sugar: 1g; Sodium:

250mg; Potassium: 120mg; Phosphorus: 120mg

Egg Drop Soup

Degree of Difficulty: ★★☆☆☆

Preparation time: five mins

Cooking time: ten mins

Servings: four

Ingredients:

- quarter teacup minced fresh chives
- four teacups unsalted vegetable stock
- 4 whisked eggs

Directions:

1. Pour unsalted vegetable stock into the oven set over high temp. Raise towards a boil. Lower temp.
2. Pour in the eggs. Stir till ribbons form into the soup.
3. Turn off the heat instantly. The residual heat will cook eggs through.
4. Cool slightly prior to ladling the anticipated quantity into individual bowls. Garnish with a pinch of parsley, if using.
5. Serve instantly.

Per serving: Calories: 73kcal; Fat: 3g; Carbs: 1g; Protein: 7g; Sugar: 6g; Sodium: 391mg; Potassium: 53mg; Phosphorus: 36mg

Apple Cinnamon Overnight Oats

Degree of Difficulty: ★☆☆☆☆

Preparation time: five mins

Cooking time: zero mins

Servings: 1

Ingredients:

- half teacup rolled oats
- half teacup low-fat milk or an almond milk
- quarter teacup cubed apples
- one tbsp severed almonds
- one tbsp ground flaxseed
- half tsp cinnamon
- one tsp honey (optional)

Directions:

1. Inside a jar or container with a cover, blend the rolled oats, milk, cubed apples, severed almonds, ground flaxseed, cinnamon, and honey (if anticipated).
2. Stir well to blend.
3. Cover the jar/container and put in the fridge for almost four hrs or overnight, letting the oats to soften and absorb the liquid.
4. Stir the overnight oats prior to serving to distribute the components.
5. Serve cooled.

Per serving: Calories: 280kcal; Fat: 12g; Carbs: 35g; Protein: 10g; Sugar: 8g; Sodium: 70mg; Potassium: 320mg; Phosphorus: 260m

Lunch Recipes

Grilled Turkey Burgers

Degree of Difficulty: ★★☆☆

Preparation time: fifteen mins

Cooking time: twelve mins

Servings: four

Ingredients:

- one lb. ground turkey
- one small onion, finely severed
- one piece garlic, crushed
- one tbsp Worcestershire sauce
- one tsp dried oregano
- Salt and pepper as required
- Lettuce leaves, sliced tomatoes, and whole-wheat buns for serving

Directions:

1. Warm up the grill to middling temp..
2. Inside a container, blend ground turkey, severed onion, crushed garlic, Worcestershire sauce, dried oregano, salt, and pepper. Mix thoroughly.
3. Split the mixture into four similar parts then shape them into burger patties.
4. Grill the turkey burgers for around five to six mins per side, or till cooked through.
5. Serve the burgers on whole-wheat buns with lettuce leaves and sliced tomatoes.

Per serving: Calories: 250kcal; Fat: 9gm; Carbs: 21g; Protein: 22g; Sugar: 3gm; Sodium: 140mg; Potassium: 310mg; Phosphorus: 210mg

Quinoa and Vegetable Stir-Fry

Degree of Difficulty: ★★☆☆

Preparation time: fifteen mins

Cooking time: fifteen mins

Servings: four

Ingredients:

- one teacup quinoa
- 2 cups low-sodium vegetable broth
- one tbsp olive oil
- one small onion, severed
- two pieces garlic, crushed
- one small zucchini, cut
- one small yellow squash, cut
- one red bell pepper, cut
- one teacup broccoli florets
- two tbsps low-sodium soy sauce
- one tsp sesame oil
- Salt and pepper as required

Directions:

1. Give the quinoa a quick wash in some ice water.

2. Raise the vegetable broth to a boil in the saucepot you have chosen to use. Put the quinoa after it has been washed, and lower the temp. to a low setting. Protect and continue to boil across low heat for approximately fifteen mins, or until the quinoa is cooked and all of the liquid has been consumed.

3. Over a middling temp., warm the olive oil in the enormous griddle you have. After adding the onion and garlic, continue cooking till the mixture becomes scented.

4. Include the zucchini, yellow squash, red bell pepper, and broccoli florets to the griddle. Stir-fry for around five to seven mins, or till the vegetables are soft-crisp.

5. Stir in the cooked quinoa, low-sodium soy sauce, sesame oil, salt, and pepper. Cook for an additional two-three mins, blending thoroughly to blend.

6. Serve warm.

Per serving: Calories: 220kcal; Fat: 6g; Carbs: 36g; Protein: 8g; Sugar: 4g; Sodium: 220mg; Potassium: 320mg; Phosphorus: 150mg

Shrimp Stir-Fry

Degree of Difficulty: ★★☆☆☆
Preparation time: ten mins
Cooking time: ten mins
Servings: 2

Ingredients:

- half lb. shrimp, skinned and deveined
- one tbsp olive oil
- one small onion, severed
- one piece garlic, crushed
- one small carrot, thinly cut
- one small bell pepper, cut
- one teacup snap peas
- two tbsps low-sodium soy sauce
- one tbsp honey (optional)
- Salt and pepper as required

Directions:

1. Warm olive oil in your griddle in a middling temp. Include the onion and garlic then sauté till fragrant.

2. Include the shrimp to the griddle then cook for around two-three mins on all sides till they go pink and opaque. Take out the shrimp from the griddle then put away.

3. Inside the similar griddle, include the carrot, bell pepper, and snap peas. Stir-fry for around four to five mins till the vegetables are soft-crisp.

4. Inside a small container, whisk collectively low-sodium soy sauce and honey (if using). Pour the sauce across the vegetables then stir well.

5. Place the cooked shrimp back to the griddle then throw to cover everything uniformly with the sauce.

6. Season with salt and pepper as required.

7. Serve the shrimp stir-fry as a light and protein-packed lunch.

Per serving: Calories: 220kcal; Fat: 7g; Carbs: 16g; Protein: 23g; Sugar: 10g; Sodium: 300mg; Potassium: 250mg; Phosphorus: 120mg

Greek Salad with Grilled Chicken

Degree of Difficulty: ★★☆☆

Preparation time: fifteen mins

Cooking time: fifteen mins

Servings: two

Ingredients:

- two boneless, skinless chicken breasts
- four teacups mixed salad greens
- one small cucumber, cubed
- half teacup cherry tomatoes, halved
- quarter teacup cut red onion
- quarter teacup Kalamata olives
- two tbsps crumbled feta cheese
- two tbsps extra-virgin olive oil
- one tbsp red wine vinegar
- one tsp dried oregano
- Salt and pepper as required

Directions:

1. Warm up the grill to medium-high temp.
2. Flavour the chicken breasts with pepper, salt & dried oregano.
3. Grill the chicken breasts for around 6-8 minutes per side, or till cooked through.

Let them rest for a couple of mins prior to slicing.

4. Inside a big container, blend the mixed salad greens, cubed cucumber, cherry tomatoes, cut red onion, and Kalamata olives.
5. Inside your small container, whisk collectively extra-virgin olive oil, red wine vinegar, dried oregano, salt and pepper to create the dressing.
6. Place the dressing to the salad and throw to cover all uniformly.
7. Split the salad into two plates and top each with the cut grilled chicken.
8. Spray crumbled feta cheese on top.
9. Serve the Greek salad with grilled chicken as a refreshing and protein-rich lunch option.

Per serving: Calories: 280kcal; Fat: 15g; Carbs: 10g; Protein: 28g; Sugar: 4g; Sodium: 200mg; Potassium: 240mg; Phosphorus: 100mg

Cauliflower Rice Stir-Fry with Chicken

Degree of Difficulty: ★★☆☆

Preparation time: ten mins

Cooking time: fifteen mins

Servings: 2

Ingredients:

- 2 boneless, skinless chicken breasts, that is cut into bite-sized parts

- two teacups cauliflower rice
- one tbsp olive oil
- one small onion, severed
- two pieces garlic, crushed
- one small carrot, thinly cut
- one teacup snap peas
- two tbsps low-sodium soy sauce
- Salt and pepper as required

Directions:

1. Inside your griddle, heat olive oil across middling temp. Place the severed onion and crushed garlic and sauté till fragrant.

2. Include the chicken breast pieces to the griddle and cook for around four to five mins till they are cooked through. Take out the chicken from the griddle then put away.

3. Inside the similar griddle, include the cauliflower rice, cut carrot, and snap peas. Stir-fry for around four to five mins till the vegetables are soft-crisp.

4. Return the cooked chicken to the griddle and include low-sodium soy sauce. Stir thoroughly to blend all the components.

5. Flavour with salt and pepper as required.

6. Serve the cauliflower rice stir-fry with chicken hot.

Per serving: Calories: 250kcal; Fat: 9g; Carbs: 12g; Protein: 28g; Sugar: 5g; Sodium: 200mg; Potassium: 280mg; Phosphorus: 180mg

Baked Salmon with Herbs

Degree of Difficulty: ★★☆☆☆

Preparation time: ten mins

Cooking time: twenty mins

Servings: two

Ingredients:

- two salmon fillets
- one tbsp olive oil
- one tsp dried dill
- one tsp dried parsley
- Salt and pepper as required

Directions:

1. Warm up the oven to 375°F.

2. Bring the salmon fillets onto a baking tray covered with parchment paper.

3. Spray the salmon with olive oil then spray with dried dill, dried parsley, salt, and pepper.

4. Bake in the oven for around fifteen-twenty mins, or 'til the salmon is cooked through and flakes simply with a fork.

Per serving: Calories: 300kcal; Fat: 18g; Carbs: 0g; Protein: 33g; Sugar: 0gm; Sodium: 70mg; Potassium: 270mg; Phosphorus: 130mg

Baked Cod with Lemon and Herbs

Degree of Difficulty: ★★☆☆☆

Preparation time: ten mins

Cooking time: twenty mins

Servings: 2

Ingredients:

- two cod fillets
- 1 lemon, juiced and zested
- one tbsp olive oil
- one tsp dried herbs (thyme, rosemary, or dill)
- Salt and pepper as required

Directions:

1. Warm up the oven to 375°F.
2. Bring the cod fillets on a baking sheet lined with parchment paper.
3. Inside your small container, whisk collectively lemon juice, lemon zest, olive oil, dried herbs, salt, and pepper.
4. Pour the marinade over the cod fillets and make sure they are covered uniformly.
5. Bake in the oven for around fifteen-twenty mins, or 'til the fish is opaque and flakes simply with a fork.
6. Serve the baked cod with lemon and herbs hot.

Per serving: Calories: 200kcal; Fat: 7g; Carbs: 2g; Protein: 32g; Sugar: 0g; Sodium: 100mg; Potassium: 250mg; Phosphorus: 120mg

Spinach and Feta Stuffed Chicken Breast

Degree of Difficulty: ★★★★☆

Preparation time: fifteen mins

Cooking time: twenty-five mins

Servings: 2

Ingredients:

- 2 boneless, skinless chicken breasts
- one teacup fresh spinach leaves
- quarter teacup crumbled feta cheese
- one piece garlic, crushed
- one tsp olive oil
- Salt and pepper as required

Directions:

1. Warm up the oven to 375°F.
2. Butterfly the chicken breasts by cutting horizontally through the center, but not all the way through, to create a pocket.
3. In your griddle, warm the olive oil in a middling temp. Include the crushed garlic and sauté till fragrant.
4. Place the fresh spinach leaves to the griddle and cook till wilted. Take out from heat.
5. Stuff the spinach and feta cheese into the pockets of the chicken breasts.
6. Flavour the stuffed chicken breasts with salt and pepper.

7. Warm a separate griddle inside a medium-high temp. then sear the chicken breasts for 2-3 mins on all sides till browned.

8. Bring the chicken breasts to a baking dish and bake in the oven for around fifteen-twenty mins, or till the chicken is cooked through.

9. Let the chicken to rest for a couple of mins prior to serving.

Per serving: Calories: 240kcal; Fat: 9gm; Carbs: 2g; Protein: 36g; Sugar: 0g; Sodium: 130mg; Potassium: 270mg; Phosphorus: 180mg

Caprese Salad with Grilled Chicken

Degree of Difficulty: ★★★★★

Preparation time: ten mins

Cooking time: fifteen mins

Servings: two

Ingredients:

- 2 boneless, skinless chicken breasts
- one tbsp olive oil
- 2 medium tomatoes, cut
- half teacup fresh mozzarella cheese, cut
- quarter teacup fresh basil leaves
- one tbsp balsamic glaze
- Salt and pepper as required

Directions:

1. Warm up the grill to medium-high temp.

2. Flavour the chicken breasts with salt & pepper.

3. Grill the chicken breasts for around 6-8 minutes per side, or till cooked through. Allow them to relax for a couple of mins prior to slicing.

4. Inside a container, arrange the cut tomatoes and fresh mozzarella cheese.

5. Top the tomatoes and cheese with fresh basil leaves.

6. Spray the balsamic glaze over the salad.

7. Slice the grilled chicken breasts and place them on top of the salad.

8. Flavour with salt and pepper as required.

9. Serve the Caprese salad with grilled chicken as a light and flavorful lunch option.

Per serving: Calories: 280kcal; Fat: 14g; Carbs: 6g; Protein: 32g; Sugar: 4g; Sodium: 200mg; Potassium: 330mg; Phosphorus: 220mg

Lentil and Vegetable Curry

Degree of Difficulty: ★★★★☆

Preparation time: fifteen mins

Cooking time: thirty-five mins

Servings: 4

Ingredients:

- one teacup dried green lentils
- one tbsp olive oil
- one small onion, severed
- two pieces garlic, crushed
- one small carrot, cubed

- one small bell pepper, cubed
- one small zucchini, cubed
- one tbsp curry powder
- one tsp ground cumin
- half tsp ground coriander
- quarter tsp turmeric
- one teacup low-sodium vegetable broth
- one teacup coconut milk (light or full-fat)
- Salt and pepper as required
- Fresh cilantro for garnish (optional)

Directions:

1. Wash the dried lentils under cold water.

2. Inside a saucepot, raise water towards a boil. Include the washed lentils then cook for around fifteen-twenty mins, or till they are soft. Drain and put away.

3. In your different pot, warm the olive oil in a middling temp. Place the severed onion and crushed garlic and sauté till fragrant.

4. Include the cubed carrot, bell pepper, and zucchini to the pot. Cook for around five to seven mins, mixing irregularly.

5. Stir in the curry powder, ground cumin, ground coriander, and turmeric. Cook for extra min to toast the spices.

6. Pour in the low-sodium vegetable broth and coconut milk. Stir thoroughly to blend.

7. Include the cooked lentils to the pot then simmer for around ten-fifteen mins to let the flavors to meld.

8. Flavour with salt and pepper as required.

9. Garnish with fresh cilantro, if anticipated.

10. Serve the lentil and vegetable curry hot with rice or naan bread.

Per serving: Calories: 280kcal; Fat: 10g; Carbs: 35g; Protein: 12g; Sugar: 6g; Sodium: 100mg; Potassium: 320mg; Phosphorus: 180mg

Spinach and Mushroom Stuffed Chicken Breast

Degree of Difficulty: ★★★☆☆

Preparation time: fifteen mins

Cooking time: twenty-five mins

Servings: 2

Ingredients:

- 2 boneless, skinless chicken breasts
- one teacup fresh spinach leaves
- half teacup cut mushrooms
- one piece garlic, crushed
- one tsp olive oil
- Salt and pepper as required

Directions:

1. Warm up the oven to 375°F.

2. Butterfly the chicken breasts by cutting horizontally through the center, but not all the way through, to create a pocket.

3. In your griddle, warm the olive oil inside a middling temp. Include the crushed garlic and sauté till fragrant.

4. Include the fresh spinach leaves and cut mushrooms to the griddle. Cook till the

spinach is wilted and the mushrooms are soft. Take out from fire.

5. Stuff the spinach and mushroom mixture into the pockets of the chicken breasts.

6. Flavour the stuffed chicken breasts with salt and pepper.

7. Warm a separate griddle in a medium-high temp. and sear the chicken breasts for two-three mins on all sides till browned.

8. Bring the chicken breasts to a baking dish and bake in the oven for around fifteen-twenty mins, or till the chicken is cooked through.

9. Let the chicken to rest for a couple of mins prior to serving.

Per serving: Calories: 220kcal; Fat: 7g; Carbs: 2g; Protein: 36g; Sugar: 0g; Sodium: 100mg; Potassium: 270mg; Phosphorus: 190mg

Quinoa and Black Bean Salad

Degree of Difficulty: ★★☆☆☆

Preparation time: fifteen mins

Cooking time: twenty mins

Servings: four

Ingredients:

- one teacup cooked quinoa
- one tin (fifteen oz.) black beans (washed & drained)
- one teacup cubed tomatoes
- half teacup cubed cucumber
- quarter teacup severed fresh cilantro
- two tbsps lime juice
- one tbsp olive oil
- one piece garlic, crushed
- Salt and pepper as required

Directions:

1. Inside a big container, blend the cooked quinoa, washed and drained black beans, cubed tomatoes, cubed cucumber, and severed fresh cilantro.

2. Inside your small container, whisk collectively lime juice, olive oil, crushed garlic, salt & pepper to form the dressing.

3. Transfer the dressing across the quinoa and black bean mixture. Throw well to cover all uniformly.

4. Allow the salad sit for a couple of mins to allow the flavors to meld.

5. Serve the quinoa and black bean salad cooled or at room temperature.

Per serving: Calories: 240kcal; Fat: 5gm; Carbs: 40g; Protein: 10gm; Sugar: 3g; Sodium: 200mg; Potassium: 230mg; Phosphorus: 180mg

Grilled Lemon Herb Tofu

Degree of Difficulty: ★★☆☆☆

Preparation time: ten mins

Cooking time: ten mins

Servings: two

Ingredients:

- 8 ounces extra-firm tofu, drained then cut into cubes
- one lemon, juiced
- one tbsp olive oil
- one tsp dried herbs (thyme, rosemary, or oregano)
- Salt and pepper as required

Directions:

1. Warm up the grill to medium-high temp.
2. Inside your container, whisk collectively lemon juice, olive oil, dried herbs, salt, and pepper.
3. Include the tofu cubes to the marinade then throw gently to cover.
4. Thread the tofu cubes onto skewers.
5. Grill the tofu skewers for around three to four mins per side, or till the tofu is lightly browned and warmed over.
6. Take out the tofu from the skewers and serve hot.

Per serving: Calories: 180kcal; Fat: 10gm; Carbs: 7g; Protein: 18g; Sugar: 1g; Sodium: 15mg; Potassium: 260mg; Phosphorus: 350mg

Grilled Vegetable Skewers

Degree of Difficulty: ★★☆☆☆
Preparation time: fifteen mins
Cooking time: ten mins
Servings: four
Ingredients:

- one small zucchini, cut
- one small yellow squash, cut
- one small eggplant, cubed
- one small red onion, cut into wedges
- one bell pepper, cut into chunks
- 8 cherry tomatoes
- two tbsps olive oil
- one tsp dried herbs (thyme, rosemary, or oregano)
- Salt and pepper as required

Directions:

1. Warm up the grill to medium-high temp.
2. Inside a container, throw the cut zucchini, cut yellow squash, cubed eggplant, red onion wedges, bell pepper chunks, and cherry tomatoes with olive oil, dried herbs, salt, and pepper.
3. Thread the vegetables onto skewers, alternating the different vegetables.
4. Grill the vegetable skewers for around four to five mins per side, or 'til the vegetables are soft and mildly overdone.
5. Take the skewers from the grill and serve hot.

Per serving: Calories: 120kcal; Fat: 8g; Carbs: 12g; Protein: 2gm; Sugar: 6g; Sodium: 5mg; Potassium: 370mg; Phosphorus: 70mg

Tofu Stir-Fry with Vegetables

Degree of Difficulty: ★★☆☆☆
Preparation time: fifteen mins

Cooking time: ten mins

Servings: 2

Ingredients:

- 8 ounces firm tofu, drained and cubed
- one tbsp low-sodium soy sauce
- one tbsp sesame oil
- one tbsp olive oil
- one small onion, cut
- one bell pepper, cut
- one small zucchini, cut
- one teacup snap peas
- two pieces garlic, crushed
- one tsp grated ginger
- Salt and pepper as required

Directions:

1. Inside a container, marinate the cubed tofu in low-sodium soy sauce for a couple of mins.

2. Heat sesame oil & olive oil in a griddle or wok at medium-high temp.

3. Include the cut onion, cut bell pepper, cut zucchini, snap peas, crushed garlic, and grated ginger to the griddle. Stir-fry for around four to five mins till the vegetables are soft-crisp.

4. Push the vegetables to one side of the griddle and include the marinated tofu to the other side. Cook for around two-three mins till the tofu is warmed over.

5. Mix the tofu with the vegetables in the griddle.

6. Flavour with salt and pepper as required.

7. Serve the tofu stir-fry with vegetables hot at rice or noodles.

Per serving: Calories: 230kcal; Fat: 13g; Carbs: 15g; Protein: 14g; Sugar: 6g; Sodium: 250mg; Potassium: 300mg; Phosphorus: 280mg

Grilled Shrimp Skewers with Lemon Garlic Sauce

Degree of Difficulty: ★★☆☆☆

Preparation time: fifteen mins

Cooking time: eight mins

Servings: 2

Ingredients:

- half lb. shrimp, skinned and deveined
- one tbsp olive oil
- two pieces garlic, crushed
- one lemon, juiced and zested
- one tbsp severed fresh parsley
- Salt and pepper as required
- Lemon Garlic Sauce:
- two tbsps low-fat Greek yogurt
- one tbsp lemon juice
- one piece garlic, crushed
- Salt and pepper as required

Directions:

1. Warm up the grill to medium-high temp.

2. Inside your container, blend the skinned and deveined shrimp, olive oil, crushed garlic, lemon juice, lemon zest, severed

fresh parsley, salt, and pepper. Mix thoroughly to cover the shrimp.

3. Thread the shrimp onto skewers.

4. Grill the shrimp skewers for around three to four mins on all sides, or till they turn pink and opaque.

5. Inside a distinct small container, whisk collectively low-fat Greek yogurt, lemon juice, crushed garlic, salt, and pepper to create the lemon garlic sauce.

6. Serve the grilled shrimp skewers with the lemon garlic sauce on the side.

7. Enjoy as a protein-rich and flavorful lunch option.

Per serving: Calories: 180kcal; Fat: 7g; Carbs: 4g; Protein: 24g; Sugar: 1g; Sodium: 220mg; Potassium: 210mg; Phosphorus: 170mg

Tuna Salad Lettuce Wraps

Degree of Difficulty: ★☆☆☆☆

Preparation time: ten mins

Cooking time: zero mins

Servings: two

Ingredients:

- 2 cans (5 ounces each) water-packed tuna, drained
- two tbsps low-fat mayonnaise
- one tbsp Dijon mustard
- one stalk celery, finely severed
- 2 green onions, cut

- Salt and pepper as required
- Lettuce leaves for wrapping

Directions:

1. Inside a container, blend the drained water-packed tuna, low-fat mayonnaise, Dijon mustard, finely severed celery, cut green onions, salt, and pepper. Mix thoroughly.

2. Spoon the tuna salad onto lettuce leaves and wrap them up.

3. Serve as a light and low-carb lunch option.

Per serving: Calories: 180kcal; Fat: 5g; Carbs: 3g; Protein: 30g; Sugar: 1g; Sodium: 250mg; Potassium: 120mg; Phosphorus: 280mg

Vegetarian Gobi Curry

Degree of Difficulty: ★★★★☆

Preparation time: twenty mins

Cooking time: fifteen mins

Servings: two

Ingredients:

- one teacups cauliflower florets
- one tbsp unsalted butter
- 1/2 medium dry white onion, thinly severed
- quarter teacup green peas
- half tsp fresh ginger, severed
- quarter tsp turmeric
- half tsp garam masala
- 1/8 tsp cayenne pepper

- half tbsp water

Directions:

1. Heat your griddle across middling temp. with the butter and sauté the onions till caramelized.
2. Include the ginger, garam masala, turmeric, and cayenne. Include the cauliflower and peas then stir well.
3. Include the water and cover with a lid. Adjust to low heat and let it cook for ten mins. Serve with white rice.

Per serving: Calories: 31lkcal; Fat: 6.4g; Carbs: 7.3g; Protein: 2.1g; Sugar: 4g; Sodium: 39.3mg; Potassium: 209.5mg; Phosphorus: 42mg

Beef Brisket

Degree of Difficulty: ★★★★☆

Preparation time: ten mins

Cooking time: three and half hrs

Servings: six

Ingredients:

- 12 ounces trimmed chuck roast
- two pieces garlic
- one tbsp thyme
- one tbsp rosemary
- one tbsp mustard
- quarter teacup extra virgin olive oil
- one tsp black pepper
- one cubed onion
- one teacup, skinned and cut carrots

- two teacups low salt stock

Directions:

1. Warm up the oven to 300 deg. F.
2. Soak vegetables in warm water.
3. Make a paste by mixing together the thyme, mustard, rosemary, and garlic. Then mix in the oil and pepper.
4. Include the beef to the dish.
5. Pour the solution over the beef into a dish.
6. Place the vegetables onto the lower part of the baking dish around the beef.
7. Cover and roast for 3 hours, or till soft.
8. Uncover the dish and start to cook for thirty mins in the oven.
9. Serve.

Per serving: Calories: 303kcal; Fat: 25g; Carbs: 7g; Protein: 18g; Sugar: 8g; Sodium: 44mg; Potassium: 246mg; Phosphorus: 276mg

Greek-Style Roasted Vegetables

Degree of Difficulty: ★★☆☆☆

Preparation time: ten mins

Cooking time: twenty-five mins

Servings: four

Ingredients:

- one small eggplant, cubed
- one small zucchini, cubed
- one small red bell pepper, cubed
- 1small yellow bell pepper, cubed

- one small red onion, cut
- two tbsps olive oil
- one tsp dried oregano
- half tsp dried thyme
- Salt and pepper as required
- Lemon wedges for serving

Directions:

1. Warm up the oven to 425°F.

2. Inside a big baking tray, blend the cubed eggplant, cubed zucchini, cubed red bell pepper, cubed yellow bell pepper, and cut red onion.

3. Spray olive oil across the vegetables then spray with dried oregano, dried thyme, salt, and pepper. Throw well to cover all the vegetables uniformly.

4. Disperse the vegetables out in an even layer in the baking dish.

5. Roast in the oven for around twenty to twenty-five mins, or 'til the vegetables are soft and mildly browned, stirring once or twice during cooking.

6. Serve the Greek-style roasted vegetables hot with lemon wedges on the side.

Per serving: Calories: 120kcal; Fat: 7g; Carbs: 15g; Protein: 2g; Sugar: 8gm; Sodium: 10mg; Potassium: 240mg; Phosphorus: 60mg

Baked Pork Chops with Rosemary

Degree of Difficulty: ★★☆☆☆

Preparation time: ten mins

Cooking time: twenty-five mins

Servings: two

Ingredients:

- two boneless pork chops
- one tbsp olive oil
- one tsp dried rosemary
- half tsp garlic powder
- Salt and pepper as required

Directions:

1. Warm up the oven to 375°F.

2. Warm the olive oil in your griddle in a medium-high temp.

3. Flavour the pork chops with dried rosemary, garlic powder, salt, and pepper.

4. Sear the pork chops in your griddle for around two-three mins on all sides, or till browned.

5. Bring the pork chops to a baking tray and bake in the oven for around fifteen-twenty mins, or till cooked through.

6. Let the pork chops cool for a couple of mins prior to serving.

Per serving: Calories: 280kcal; Fat: 14g; Carbs: 0gm; Protein: 36g; Sugar: 0g; Sodium: 90mg; Potassium: 300mg; Phosphorus: 300mg

Broccoli and Chicken Stir-Fry

Degree of Difficulty: ★★☆☆☆

Preparation time: ten mins

Cooking time: fifteen mins

Servings: 2

Ingredients:

- 2 boneless, skinless chicken breasts, thinly cut
- one tbsp olive oil
- two teacups broccoli florets
- one small carrot, thinly cut
- half teacup cut bell peppers
- two pieces garlic, crushed
- two tbsps low-sodium soy sauce
- one tbsp oyster sauce (optional)
- Salt and pepper as required

Directions:

1. Warm olive oil in your griddle or wok at medium-high temp. Include the crushed garlic and sauté till fragrant.

2. Include the cut chicken breasts to the griddle and stir-fry for around four to five mins till they are cooked through. Take out the chicken from the griddle then put away.

3. Inside the similar griddle, place the broccoli florets, cut carrot, and cut bell peppers. Stir-fry for around four to five mins till the vegetables are soft-crisp.

4. Return the cooked chicken to the griddle and include low-sodium soy sauce and oyster sauce (if required). Stir thoroughly to blend the entire components.

5. Flavour with salt and pepper as required.

6. Serve the broccoli and chicken stir-fry hot as a nutritious and flavorful lunch.

Per serving: Calories: 280kcal; Fat: 10g; Carbs: 12g; Protein: 34g; Sugar: 4g; Sodium: 200mg; Potassium: 280mg; Phosphorus: 220mg

Roasted Salmon with Dill

Degree of Difficulty: ★★☆☆☆

Preparation time: ten mins

Cooking time: fifteen mins

Servings: two

Ingredients:

- two salmon fillets
- one tbsp olive oil
- one tbsp fresh dill, severed
- one lemon, cut
- Salt and pepper as required

Directions:

1. Warm up the oven to 425°F.

2. Bring the salmon fillets onto a baking tray covered with parchment paper.

3. Spray the olive oil in the salmon fillets.

4. Spray the fresh dill, salt, and pepper over the salmon.

5. Place a few slices of lemon on top of each salmon fillet.

6. Bake in the oven for around twelve-fifteen mins, or 'til the salmon is cooked through and flakes simply with a fork.

7. Serve the roasted salmon with dill hot.

Per serving: Calories: 300kcal; Fat: 16g; Carbs: 0g; Protein: 36g; Sugar: 0g; Sodium: 120mg; Potassium: 250mg; Phosphorus: 120mg

Dinner Recipes

Turkey Meatballs with Marinara Sauce

Degree of Difficulty: ★★☆☆☆

Preparation time: fifteen mins

Cooking time: twenty-five mins

Servings: four

Ingredients:

- one lb. ground turkey
- quarter teacup bread crumbs (low-sodium if available)
- quarter teacup grated Parmesan cheese
- quarter teacup severed fresh parsley
- 1 egg
- two pieces garlic, crushed
- half tsp dried oregano
- half tsp dried basil
- Salt and pepper as required
- two teacups low-sodium marinara sauce

Directions:

1. Warm up the oven to 375°F.
2. Inside your container, blend the ground turkey, bread crumbs, Parmesan cheese, parsley, egg, crushed garlic, dried oregano, dried basil, salt, and pepper.
3. Shape the solution into meatballs then place them onto a baking tray.
4. Bake for twenty to twenty-five mins or 'til the meatballs are cooked through.
5. Inside a saucepot, warm the marinara sauce across middling temp. till warmed.
6. Serve the turkey meatballs with the marinara sauce.

Per serving: Calories: 250kcal; Fat: 8gm; Carbs: 15g; Protein: 28g; Sugar: 6g; Sodium: 200mg; Potassium: 350mg; Phosphorus: 260mg

Vegetable Stir-Fry with Shrimp

Degree of Difficulty: ★★☆☆☆

Preparation time: fifteen mins

Cooking time: ten mins

Servings: four

Ingredients:

- one lb. shrimp, skinned and deveined
- two teacups mixed vegetables (e.g., broccoli, bell peppers, carrots, snap peas)
- two pieces garlic, crushed
- two tbsps low-sodium soy sauce
- one tbsp sesame oil
- one tsp cornstarch (optional for thickening the sauce)
- Salt and pepper as required
- Cooked brown rice for serving

Directions:

1. Heat the sesame oil in your huge griddle or wok at medium-high temp.

2. Include the crushed garlic and stir-fry for one min.

3. Include the shrimp then stir-fry for two-three mins till they go pink and opaque.

4. Include the mixed vegetables to the griddle then stir-fry for an additional three to four mins till they are crisp-soft.

5. Inside your small container, whisk collectively the soy sauce and cornstarch (if using) till even.

6. Transfer the sauce across the shrimp and vegetables, and stir-fry for one min 'til the sauce denses mildly.

7. Flavour with salt and pepper as required.

8. Serve the stir-fry over cooked brown rice.

Per serving: Calories: 220kcal; Fat: 5g; Carbs: 15g; Protein: 28g; Sugar: 4g; Sodium: 300mg; Potassium: 380mg; Phosphorus: 250mg

Lemon Garlic Roasted Chicken Thighs

Degree of Difficulty: ★★☆☆☆

Preparation time: ten mins

Cooking time: forty mins

Servings: four

Ingredients:

- four chicken thighs, bone-in and skin-on
- two tbsps olive oil
- two pieces garlic, crushed
- one lemon, juiced and zested
- one tsp dried thyme

- Salt and pepper as required

Directions:

1. Warm up the oven to 400°F.

2. Inside your small container, blend the olive oil, crushed garlic, lemon juice, lemon zest, dried thyme, salt, and pepper.

3. Bring the chicken thighs in a baking tray and pour the lemon garlic solution over them, making sure to cover them uniformly.

4. Roast in the oven for thirty-five to forty mins or till the chicken is cooked through and the skin is crispy.

5. Serve the chicken thighs with your choice of side dishes.

Per serving: Calories: 300kcal; Fat: 20g; Carbs: 1g; Protein: 28g; Sugar: 0g; Sodium: 150mg; Potassium: 320mg; Phosphorus: 250mg

Beef and Vegetable Stir-Fry

Degree of Difficulty: ★★☆☆☆

Preparation time: fifteen mins

Cooking time: ten mins

Servings: four

Ingredients:

- one lb. beef sirloin, thinly cut
- two teacups mixed vegetables (e.g., bell peppers, broccoli, carrots, snap peas)
- two pieces garlic, crushed
- two tbsps low-sodium soy sauce

- one tbsp sesame oil
- one tsp cornstarch (optional for thickening the sauce)
- Salt and pepper as required
- Cooked brown rice for serving

Directions:

1. Heat the sesame oil in your huge griddle or wok at medium-high temp.
2. Include the crushed garlic and stir-fry for one min.
3. Place the cut beef to the griddle and stir-fry for two-three mins till it's browned.
4. Include the mixed vegetables to the griddle then stir-fry for an additional three to four mins till they are crisp-soft.
5. Inside your small container, whisk collectively the soy sauce and cornstarch (if using) till even.
6. Pour the sauce over the beef & vegetables, and stir-fry for one min 'til the sauce denses mildly.
7. Flavour with salt and pepper as required.
8. Serve the stir-fry over cooked brown rice.

Per serving: Calories: 300kcal; Fat: 12g; Carbs: 15g; Protein: 30g; Sugar: 4g; Sodium: 200mg; Potassium: 300mg; Phosphorus: 160mg

Beer Pork Ribs

Degree of Difficulty: ★★★★☆

Preparation time: ten mins

Cooking time: 8 hours

Servings: two

Ingredients:

- four pounds of pork ribs, cut into two units/racks
- 18 oz. of root beer
- two pieces of garlic, crushed
- two tbsps of onion powder
- two tbsps of vegetable oil (optional)

Directions:

1. Wrap the pork ribs with vegetable oil and place one unit on the lower part of your slow cooker with half of the crushed garlic and the onion powder.
2. Place the other rack on top with the rest of the garlic and onion powder.
3. Pour over the root beer and cover the lid.
4. Let simmer for 8 hours on low heat.
5. Take off and finish optionally in a grilling pan for a nice sear.

Per serving: Calories: 301kcal; Fat: 18g; Carbs: 36g; Protein: 21g; Sugar: 4g; Sodium: 329mg; Potassium: 100mg; Phosphorus: 109 mg

Baked Cod with Roasted Vegetables

Degree of Difficulty: ★★☆☆☆

Preparation time: ten mins

Cooking time: twenty-five mins

Servings: four

Ingredients:

- four cod fillets
- one zucchini, cut
- one yellow squash, cut
- one red bell pepper, cut
- one red onion, cut
- two tbsps olive oil
- one tsp dried oregano
- Salt and pepper as required

Directions:

1. Warm up the oven to 400°F.
2. Bring the cod fillets in a baking tray.
3. Inside a separate container, throw the cut zucchini, yellow squash, red bell pepper & red onion with olive oil, dried oregano, salt & pepper.
4. Place the fish fillets in the baking tray and put the veggies within a ring surrounding them.
5. Place in the oven and bake for twenty to twenty-five mins, or till the fish is fully cooked and the veggies have reached the desired consistency.

Per serving: Calories: 220kcal; Fat: 8g; Carbs: 12g; Protein: 25g; Sugar: 6g; Sodium: 100mg; Potassium: 300mg; Phosphorus: 180mg

Grilled Salmon with Herbed Quinoa

Degree of Difficulty: ★★★☆☆

Preparation time: fifteen mins

Cooking time: twenty mins

Servings: four

Ingredients:

- four salmon fillets
- one teacup quinoa
- two teacups low-sodium chicken or vegetable broth
- one tbsp severed fresh dill
- one tbsp severed fresh parsley
- Salt and pepper as required

Directions:

1. Warm up the grill to middling temp.
2. Wash the quinoa underneath cold water.
3. Inside your saucepot, raise the chicken or vegetable broth to a boil then place the quinoa.
4. Decrease temp., cover then simmer for fifteen mins or 'til the quinoa is cooked and the liquid is engrossed.
5. Pour the salmon fillets with salt & pepper, and your choice of herbs.
6. Grill the salmon for four to five mins on all sides or till cooked to your anticipated doneness.
7. Fluff the quinoa with a fork then stir in the severed dill and parsley.

Per serving: Calories: 300kcal; Fat: 12g; Carbs: 20g; Protein: 28gm; Sugar: 0g; Sodium: 150mg; Potassium: 280mg; Phosphorus: 200mg

Baked Lemon Dill Salmon

Degree of Difficulty: ★★☆☆

Preparation time: ten mins

Cooking time: twenty mins

Servings: four

Ingredients:

- four salmon fillets
- one lemon, juiced and zested
- two tbsps fresh dill, severed
- two tbsps olive oil
- Salt and pepper as required

Directions:

1. Warm up the oven to 375°F.
2. Bring the salmon fillets inside a baking tray.
3. Inside your small container, blend the lemon juice, lemon zest, fresh dill, olive oil, salt, and pepper.
4. Pour the solution over the salmon fillets, making sure they are uniformly covered.
5. Bake for fifteen-twenty mins or 'til the salmon is cooked through then flakes simply with a fork.
6. Serve the baked lemon dill salmon with a side of steamed vegetables or a salad.

Per serving: Calories: 300kcal; Fat: 18g; Carbs: 2g; Protein: 32g; Sugar: 0g; Sodium: 100mg; Potassium: 280mg; Phosphorus: 250mg

Eggplant and Tomato Casserole

Degree of Difficulty: ★★★☆

Preparation time: twenty mins

Cooking time: forty mins

Servings: four

Ingredients:

- one large eggplant, cut
- two large tomatoes, cut
- 1 onion, cut
- two pieces garlic, crushed
- two tbsps olive oil
- one tsp dried oregano
- one tsp dried basil
- Salt and pepper as required
- quarter teacup grated Parmesan cheese

Directions:

1. Warm up the oven to 375°F.
2. Warm the olive oil in your griddle in a middling temp.
3. Place the cut onion and crushed garlic to the griddle and sauté till they become translucent.
4. Take out the onion & garlic from the griddle then set them aside.
5. Inside the similar griddle, include the eggplant slices and cook for three to four mins on all sides till they become soft.
6. Oil a baking tray and arrange a layer of cooked eggplant slices at the lower part.

7. Top the eggplant with a layer of cut tomatoes, sautéed onion, and garlic solution, dried oregano, dried basil, salt, and pepper.

8. Replicate the layering till the entire components are utilized, concluding with a layer of eggplant on top.

9. Pour the grated Parmesan cheese over the top.

10. Bake for 35-forty mins or 'til the casserole is hot and bubbly.

Per serving: Calories: 180kcal; Fat: 8g; Carbs: 20g; Protein: 8g; Sugar: 10g; Sodium: 120mg; Potassium: 250mg; Phosphorus: 210mg

Baked Lemon Herb Chicken

Degree of Difficulty: ★★☆☆☆

Preparation time: ten mins

Cooking time: thirty mins

Servings: four

Ingredients:

- four boneless, skinless chicken breasts
- one lemon, juiced and zested
- one tsp dried thyme
- one tsp dried rosemary
- Salt and pepper as required

Directions:

1. Warm up the oven to 375°F.

2. Bring the chicken breasts inside a baking tray.

3. Inside your small container, blend the lemon juice, lemon zest, thyme, rosemary, salt, and pepper.

4. Pour the solution across the chicken breasts.

5. Bake for twenty-five to thirty mins or 'til the chicken is cooked through.

Per serving: Calories: 200kcal; Fat: 4g; Carbs: 3g; Protein: 38gm; Sugar: 1gm; Sodium: 100mg; Potassium: 380mg; Phosphorus: 290mg

Turkey Chili

Degree of Difficulty: ★★★☆☆

Preparation time: fifteen mins

Cooking time: forty-five mins

Servings: 6

Ingredients:

- one lb. ground turkey
- one onion, cubed
- two pieces garlic, crushed
- one bell pepper, cubed
- one tin (fourteen oz.) low-sodium cubed tomatoes
- one tin (fourteen oz.) low-sodium kidney beans, drained and washed
- one tbsp chili powder
- one tsp cumin
- half tsp paprika
- Salt and pepper as required

- Chopped fresh cilantro for garnish (optional)

Directions:

1. Inside a big pot or Dutch oven, brown the ground turkey across middling temp.

2. Include the cubed onion, crushed garlic, and cubed bell pepper to the pot, and cook 'til the vegetables are soft.

3. Stir in the cubed tomatoes, kidney beans, chili powder, cumin, paprika, salt, and pepper.

4. Raise the chili to a simmer, then lower the temp. to low and conceal the pot.

5. Allow the chili simmer for thirty-forty mins to let the flavors to meld collectively.

6. Serve the turkey chili hot, garnished with severed fresh cilantro if anticipated.

Per serving: Calories: 250kcal; Fat: 8g; Carbs: 20g; Protein: 28g; Sugar: 6gm; Sodium: 200mg; Potassium: 280mg; Phosphorus: 200mg

Shrimp and Asparagus Stir-Fry

Degree of Difficulty: ★★☆☆☆

Preparation time: fifteen mins

Cooking time: ten mins

Servings: 4

Ingredients:

- one lb. shrimp, skinned and deveined
- one bunch asparagus, trimmed then cut into 2-inch parts
- one red bell pepper, cut
- one onion, cut
- two pieces garlic, crushed
- two tbsps low-sodium soy sauce
- one tbsp sesame oil
- one tsp cornstarch (optional for thickening the sauce)
- Salt and pepper as required
- Cooked brown rice for serving

Directions:

1. Heat the sesame oil in your huge griddle or wok at medium-high temp.

2. Include the crushed garlic and stir-fry for one min.

3. Place the shrimp to the griddle and stir-fry for two-three mins till they go pink and opaque.

4. Include the asparagus, red bell pepper, and onion to the griddle and stir-fry for an additional three to four mins till the vegetables are crisp-soft.

5. Inside your small container, whisk collectively the soy sauce and cornstarch (if using) till even.

6. Transfer the sauce over the shrimp and vegetables, and stir-fry for one min 'til the sauce denses mildly.

7. Flavour with salt and pepper as required.

8. Serve the stir-fry over cooked brown rice.

Per serving: Calories: 220kcal; Fat: 5g; Carbs: 15g; Protein: 28g; Sugar: 4g; Sodium:

300mg; Potassium: 380mg; Phosphorus: 250mg

Baked Herb-Crusted White Fish

Degree of Difficulty: ★★☆☆

Preparation time: ten mins

Cooking time: fifteen mins

Servings: four

Ingredients:

- four white fish fillets (tilapia or cod)
- quarter teacup bread crumbs (low-sodium if available)
- one tbsp severed fresh parsley
- one tsp dried thyme
- one tsp dried oregano
- two tbsps olive oil
- Salt and pepper as required

Directions:

1. Warm up the oven to 400°F.
2. Inside your small container, blend the bread crumbs, severed parsley, dried thyme, dried oregano, salt, and pepper.
3. Pour the olive oil across the fish fillets, then spray the herb solution on top, pressing gently to adhere.
4. Bring the fish fillets onto a baking tray lined with parchment paper.
5. Bake for twelve-fifteen mins or 'til the fish is opaque then flakes simply with a fork.
6. Serve the herb-crusted fish with a side of steamed vegetables or a salad.

Per serving: Calories: 180kcal; Fat: 8g; Carbs: 5g; Protein: 24g; Sugar: 1g; Sodium: 120mg; Potassium: 350mg; Phosphorus: 210mg

Quinoa and Vegetable Stuffed Bell Peppers

Degree of Difficulty: ★★★☆

Preparation time: twenty mins

Cooking time: forty mins

Servings: four

Ingredients:

- 4 bell peppers (any color), tops take out and seeds take out
- one teacup cooked quinoa
- one zucchini, cubed
- one yellow squash, cubed
- one onion, cubed
- two pieces garlic, crushed
- one tbsp olive oil
- one tsp dried basil
- one tsp dried oregano
- Salt and pepper as required
- quarter teacup grated Parmesan cheese

Directions:

1. Warm up the oven to 375°F.
2. In your griddle, warm the olive oil inside a middling temp.
3. Include the cubed zucchini, yellow squash, onion, and crushed garlic to the griddle then sauté till the vegetables are soft.

4. Inside a big container, blend the cooked quinoa, sautéed vegetables, dried basil, dried oregano, salt, and pepper.

5. Stuff each bell pepper with the quinoa and vegetable solution.

6. Bring the stuffed bell peppers in a baking tray.

7. Pour the grated Parmesan cheese over the top of each pepper.

8. Bake for thirty to thirty-five mins or till the bell peppers are soft then the cheese is dissolved and mildly golden.

Per serving: Calories: 220kcal; Fat: 8g; Carbs: 30g; Protein: 8g; Sugar: 10g; Sodium: 100mg; Potassium: 350mg; Phosphorus: 260mg

Baked Chicken and Vegetable Casserole

Degree of Difficulty: ★★★☆☆

Preparation time: twenty mins

Cooking time: forty mins

Servings: four

Ingredients:

- four boneless, skinless chicken breasts
- two teacups mixed vegetables (e.g., broccoli, carrots, cauliflower)
- one onion, cut
- two pieces garlic, crushed
- one tbsp olive oil
- one teacup low-sodium chicken broth
- one tsp dried thyme
- one tsp dried rosemary
- Salt and pepper as required

Directions:

1. Warm up the oven to 375°F.

2. In your huge griddle, warm the olive oil across middling temp.

3. Place the cut onion and crushed garlic to the griddle and sauté till they become luminous.

4. Take out the onion & garlic from the griddle then put them away.

5. Inside the similar griddle, brown the chicken breasts on both sides.

6. In a greased baking tray, layer the browned chicken breasts, sautéed onion and garlic solution, mixed vegetables, dried thyme, dried rosemary, salt, and pepper.

7. Pour the chicken broth across the casserole.

8. Cover your baking tray with foil then bake for thirty to thirty-five mins.

9. Take the foil and bake for an extra five mins or till the chicken is cooked through and the vegetables are soft.

10. Serve the baked chicken and vegetable casserole hot.

Per serving: Calories: 280kcal; Fat: 8g; Carbs: 20g; Protein: 30g; Sugar: 6g; Sodium: 200mg; Potassium: 350mg; Phosphorus: 300mg

Spinach and Mushroom Omelet

Degree of Difficulty: ★★☆☆☆

Preparation time: ten mins

Cooking time: ten mins

Servings: 2

Ingredients:

4 big eggs

- one teacup fresh spinach leaves
- half teacup cut mushrooms
- quarter teacup cubed onion
- one tbsp olive oil
- Salt and pepper as required

Directions:

1. Inside a container, whisk collectively the eggs with salt and pepper.

2. Warm the olive oil in your non-stick griddle across middling temp.

3. Include the cubed onion then cut mushrooms to the griddle and sauté till they become soft.

4. Place the fresh spinach leaves to the griddle and cook till they wither.

5. Transfer the whisked eggs over the vegetables in the griddle.

6. Cook the omelet for three to four mins or till the edges are set.

7. Carefully flip the omelet over then cook for two-three mins till it's cooked through.

8. Slide the omelet onto a plate then wrap it in half.

9. Serve the spinach and mushroom omelet hot.

Per serving: Calories: 250kcal; Fat: 18g; Carbs: 6g; Protein: 16g; Sugar: 2g; Sodium: 300mg; Potassium: 350mg; Phosphorus: 300mg

Grilled Balsamic Pork Chops

Degree of Difficulty: ★★☆☆☆

Preparation time: ten mins

Cooking time: fifteen mins

Servings: 4

Ingredients:

- four boneless pork chops
- quarter teacup balsamic vinegar
- two tbsps olive oil
- two pieces garlic, crushed
- one tsp dried rosemary
- Salt and pepper as required

Directions:

1. Warm up the grill to medium-high heat.

2. Inside your small container, whisk collectively the balsamic vinegar, olive oil, crushed garlic, dried rosemary, salt, and pepper.

3. Bring the pork chops in a shallow dish then pour the balsamic marinade across them, turning to cover both sides.

4. Grill the pork chops for six to seven mins on all sides or till cooked through.

5. Allow the pork chops rest for a couple of mins prior to serving.

Per serving: Calories: 250kcal; Fat: 12g; Carbs: 3g; Protein: 30g; Sugar: 2g; Sodium: 100mg; Potassium: 320mg; Phosphorus: 280mg

Grilled Chicken and Vegetable Skewers

Degree of Difficulty: ★★☆☆☆

Preparation time: twenty mins

Cooking time: fifteen mins

Servings: four

Ingredients:

- 2 boneless, skinless chicken breasts, that cut into chunks
- one zucchini, cut
- one yellow squash, cut
- one bell pepper, cubed
- one red onion, cubed
- two tbsps olive oil
- two tbsps lemon juice
- one tsp dried oregano
- Salt and pepper as required

Directions:

1. Warm up the grill to medium-high temp.
2. Inside your container, whisk collectively the olive oil, lemon juice, dried oregano, salt, and pepper.
3. Thread the chicken chunks, zucchini slices, yellow squash slices, bell pepper pieces, and red onion pieces onto skewers, interchanging the components.
4. Brush the skewers with the marinade, making sure to cover them uniformly.
5. Grill the skewers for ten-fifteen mins, flipping irregularly, 'til the chicken is cooked through and the vegetables are soft.
6. Serve the chicken and vegetable skewers with a side of cooked quinoa or a green salad.

Per serving: Calories: 220kcal; Fat: 8g; Carbs: 15g; Protein: 28g; Sugar: 6g; Sodium: 100mg; Potassium: 350mg; Phosphorus: 300mg

Lemon Garlic Shrimp Skewers

Degree of Difficulty: ★★☆☆☆

Preparation time: fifteen mins

Cooking time: ten mins

Servings: four

Ingredients:

- one lb. shrimp, skinned and deveined
- two lemons, juiced and zested
- two pieces garlic, crushed
- two tbsps olive oil
- one tbsp severed fresh parsley
- Salt and pepper as required

Directions:

1. Warm up the grill to medium-high temp.

2. Inside your container, blend the lemon juice, lemon zest, crushed garlic, olive oil, severed parsley, salt, and pepper.

3. Thread the shrimp onto skewers.

4. Brush the lemon garlic solution across the shrimp skewers, ensuring to cover them uniformly.

5. Grill the skewers for two-three mins on all sides or till the shrimp are pink and opaque.

6. Serve the lemon garlic shrimp skewers as an appetizer or main dish.

Per serving: Calories: 150kcal; Fat: 6g; Carbs: 4g; Protein: 22g; Sugar: 0g; Sodium: 150mg; Potassium: 280mg; Phosphorus: 180mg

Baked Cod with Lemon Caper Sauce

Degree of Difficulty: ★★☆☆

Preparation time: ten mins

Cooking time: twenty mins

Servings: four

Ingredients:

- four cod fillets
- two tbsps olive oil
- one lemon, juiced and zested
- two tbsps capers, drained
- one tbsp severed fresh parsley
- Salt and pepper as required

Directions:

1. Warm up the oven to 375°F.

2. Bring the cod fillets in a baking tray.

3. Inside your small container, blend the olive oil, lemon juice, lemon zest, capers, severed parsley, salt, and pepper.

4. Pour the solution over the cod fillets, ensuring to cover them uniformly.

5. Bake for fifteen-twenty mins or 'til the cod is cooked through then flakes simply with a fork.

6. Serve the baked cod with the lemon caper sauce.

Per serving: Calories: 200kcal; Fat: 8g; Carbs: 2g; Protein: 30g; Sugar: 0g; Sodium: 200mg; Potassium: 300mg; Phosphorus: 300mg

Beef Kabobs with Pepper

Degree of Difficulty: ★★★★☆

Preparation time: five mins.

Cooking time: ten mins.

Servings: 8

Ingredients:

- one lb. beef sirloin
- half teacup vinegar
- two tbsps salad oil
- 1 medium, severed onion
- two tbsps severed fresh parsley
- quarter tsp. black pepper
- 2 cut into strips green peppers

Directions:

1. Trim the fat from the meat; then cut it into cubes of 1 and 1/2 inches each. Mix vinegar, oil, onion, parsley, and pepper in a container,

2. Put the meat in the marinade and put it away for around 2 hours; make sure to stir from occasionally.

3. Take out the meat from the marinade and alternate it on skewers instead with green pepper.

4. Brush the pepper with the marinade and broil for around ten mins 4 inches from the heat. Serve and relish your kabobs.

Per serving: Calories: 357kcal; Fat: 24g; Carbs: 0g; Protein: 5g; Sugar: 3g; Sodium: 60mg; Potassium: 305mg; Phosphorus: 349mg

Roasted Herb Chicken Thighs with Steamed Vegetables

Degree of Difficulty: ★★☆☆☆

Preparation time: fifteen mins

Cooking time: thirty-five mins

Servings: four

Ingredients:

- 4 chicken thighs, bone-in and skin-on
- two tbsps olive oil
- one tsp dried thyme
- one tsp dried rosemary
- one tsp dried sage
- Salt and pepper as required

- four teacups mixed steamed vegetables (e.g., broccoli, cauliflower, carrots)

Directions:

1. Warm up the oven to 400°F.

2. Inside your small container, blend collectively the olive oil, dried thyme, dried rosemary, dried sage, salt, and pepper.

3. Rub the herb solution over the chicken thighs, ensuring to cover them uniformly.

4. Bring the chicken thighs in a baking tray.

5. Roast in the oven for thirty to thirty-five mins or 'til the chicken is cooked across and the skin is crispy.

6. While the chicken is roasting, steam the mixed vegetables till soft.

7. Serve the roasted herb chicken thighs with the steamed vegetables.

Per serving: Calories: 350kcal; Fat: 25g; Carbs: 5g; Protein: 25g; Sugar: 2g; Sodium: 150mg; Potassium: 200mg; Phosphorus: 100mg

Turkey and Vegetable Skillet

Degree of Difficulty: ★★★☆☆

Preparation time: ten mins

Cooking time: twenty mins

Servings: 4

Ingredients:

- one lb. ground turkey
- one onion, cubed
- two pieces garlic, crushed

- one zucchini, cubed
- one yellow squash, cubed
- one bell pepper, cubed
- one tin (fourteen oz.) low-sodium cubed tomatoes
- one tsp dried basil
- one tsp dried oregano
- Salt and pepper as required

Directions:

1. Inside a big griddle, brown the ground turkey across middling temp.
2. Place the cubed onion and crushed garlic to the griddle then cook till the onion becomes luminous.
3. Stir in the cubed zucchini, yellow squash, bell pepper, cubed tomatoes (with juice), dried basil, dried oregano, salt, and pepper.
4. Simmer the turkey and vegetable solution for ten-fifteen mins, till the vegetables are soft and the flavors have melded together.
5. Serve the turkey and vegetable griddle hot.

Per serving: Calories: 220kcal; Fat: 10g; Carbs: 10g; Protein: 24g; Sugar: 6g; Sodium: 200mg; Potassium: 280mg; Phosphorus: 300mg

Snack Recipes

Rice Cake with Tuna Salad

Degree of Difficulty: ★★☆☆☆

Preparation time: ten mins

Cooking time: zero mins

Servings: four

Ingredients:

- one rice cake (low-sodium)
- quarter teacup canned tuna in water, drained
- one tbsp cubed celery
- one tbsp cubed red onion
- one tbsp plain Greek yogurt (low-fat)
- one tsp lemon juice
- Fresh parsley, severed (for garnish)

Directions:

1. Inside your container, blend collectively the drained tuna, cubed celery, cubed red onion, Greek yogurt, and lemon juice.
2. Disperse the tuna salad solution onto the rice cake.
3. Garnish with fresh severed parsley.
4. Serve instantly.

Per serving: Calories: 150kcal; Fat: 2g; Carbs: 12g; Protein: 20g; Sugar: 2g; Sodium: 100mg; Potassium: 180mg; Phosphorus: 150mg

Vegetable Crudité Platter

Degree of Difficulty: ★☆☆☆☆

Preparation time: fifteen mins

Cooking time: zero mins

Servings: four

Ingredients:

- one carrot, cut into sticks
- 1 cucumber, cut into sticks
- one bell pepper, cut
- 1 celery stalk, cut into sticks
- Cherry tomatoes
- Broccoli florets
- Low-sodium hummus (store-bought or homemade)

Directions:

1. Organize the carrot sticks, cucumber sticks, bell pepper slices, celery sticks, cherry tomatoes, and broccoli florets on a platter.
2. Serve with low-sodium hummus for dipping.

Per serving: Calories: 60kcal; Fat: 1g; Carbs: 13g; Protein: 2g; Sugar: 6g; Sodium: 30mg; Potassium: 320mg; Phosphorus: 50mg

Cottage Cheese and Fruit Bowl

Degree of Difficulty: ★☆☆☆☆

Preparation time: five mins

Cooking time: zero mins

Servings: 1

Ingredients:

- half teacup low-fat cottage cheese
- quarter teacup fresh berries (strawberries, blueberries, raspberries)
- quarter teacup cubed pineapple (fresh or canned in juice)
- one tbsp severed almonds

Directions:

1. Inside a container, blend the low-fat cottage cheese, fresh berries, cubed pineapple, and severed almonds.
2. Mix thoroughly and serve instantly.

Per serving: Calories: 180kcal; Fat: 6g; Carbs: 17g; Protein: 15gm; Sugar: 10g; Sodium: 300mg; Potassium: 220mg; Phosphorus: 160mg

Cucumber and Yogurt Dip

Degree of Difficulty: ★☆☆☆

Preparation time: ten mins

Cooking time: zero mins

Servings: four

Ingredients:

- one cucumber, grated
- one teacup plain low-fat yogurt
- two pieces garlic, crushed
- one tbsp severed fresh dill
- Salt substitute, as required
- Black pepper, as required

Directions:

1. Inside a container, blend grated cucumber, yogurt, crushed garlic, severed dill, salt substitute, and black pepper.
2. Mix thoroughly then put in the fridge for 1 hour to allow the flavors to mix.
3. Serve as a dip with low-sodium crackers or fresh vegetable sticks.

Per serving: Calories: 70kcal; Fat: 2g; Carbs: 10g; Protein: 4g; Sugar: 6g; Sodium: 50mg; Potassium: 250mg; Phosphorus: 60mg

Baked Sweet Potato Chips

Degree of Difficulty: ★★☆☆

Preparation time: ten mins

Cooking time: twenty-five mins

Servings: 2

Ingredients:

- one medium sweet potato
- one tbsp olive oil
- Salt substitute, as required
- Black pepper, as required

Directions:

1. Warm up the oven to 400°F.
2. Peel the sweet potato and slice it thinly into rounds.

3. Inside your container, throw the sweet potato slices with olive oil, salt substitute, and black pepper.

4. Bring the sweet potato slices on a baking tray in a single layer.

5. Bake in your warmed up oven for 20-25 mins or till crispy, flipping halfway through.

6. Allow to cool prior to serving.

Per serving: Calories: 150kcal; Fat: 7gm; Carbs: 21g; Protein: 2gm; Sugar: 5g; Sodium: 30mg; Potassium: 250mg; Phosphorus: 50mg

Roasted Chickpeas

Degree of Difficulty: ★★☆☆☆

Preparation time: five mins

Cooking time: thirty mins

Servings: four

Ingredients:

- one tin chickpeas, drained and washed
- one tbsp olive oil
- half tsp ground cumin
- half tsp paprika
- quarter tsp garlic powder
- Salt substitute, as required

Directions:

1. Warm up the oven to 400°F.

2. Inside a container, throw the drained and washed chickpeas with olive oil, ground cumin, paprika, garlic powder, and salt substitute.

3. Disperse the seasoned chickpeas on a baking tray in a single layer.

4. Roast in your warmed up oven for 30 mins or till crispy, mixing irregularly.

5. Allow to cool prior to serving.

Per serving: Calories: 130kcal; Fat: 4g; Carbs: 18g; Protein: 6g; Sugar: 3g; Sodium: 10mg; Potassium: 200mg; Phosphorus: 100mg

Avocado and Tomato Salad

Degree of Difficulty: ★☆☆☆☆

Preparation time: ten mins

Cooking time: zero mins

Servings: 2

Ingredients:

- one avocado, cubed
- one tomato, cubed
- quarter red onion, thinly cut
- one tbsp severed fresh cilantro
- one tbsp lime juice
- Salt substitute, as required
- Black pepper, as required

Directions:

1. Inside your container, blend the cubed avocado, cubed tomato, thinly cut red onion, severed cilantro, lime juice, salt substitute, and black pepper.

2. Gently throw to mix well.

3. Serve instantly.

Per serving: Calories: 180kcal; Fat: 15g; Carbs: 12g; Protein: 3g; Sugar: 2g; Sodium: 10mg; Potassium: 300mg; Phosphorus: 60mg

Egg Salad Lettuce Wraps

Degree of Difficulty: ★★☆☆

Preparation time: ten mins

Cooking time: ten mins

Servings: two

Ingredients:

- four large lettuce leaves (such as romaine or butter lettuce)
- 2 hard-boiled eggs, severed
- two tbsps cubed red bell pepper
- two tbsps cubed cucumber
- two tbsps plain Greek yogurt (low-fat)
- one tsp Dijon mustard
- Salt substitute, as required
- Black pepper, as required

Directions:

1. Lay out the lettuce leaves on a flat surface.
2. Inside your container, blend the severed hard-boiled eggs, cubed red bell pepper, cubed cucumber, Greek yogurt, Dijon mustard, salt substitute, and black pepper.
3. Spoon the egg salad solution onto the lettuce leaves.
4. Roll up the lettuce leaves to form wraps.
5. Secure with toothpicks if needed.
6. Serve cooled.

Per serving: Calories: 120kcal; Fat: 6g; Carbs: 6g; Protein: 11g; Sugar: 2gm; Sodium: 150mg; Potassium: 200mg; Phosphorus: 130mg

Quinoa Salad Cups

Degree of Difficulty: ★★★☆

Preparation time: fifteen mins

Cooking time: fifteen mins

Servings: four

Ingredients:

- one teacup cooked quinoa
- quarter teacup cubed cucumber
- quarter teacup cubed tomato
- quarter teacup cubed red onion
- two tbsps severed fresh parsley
- two tbsps lemon juice
- one tbsp olive oil
- Salt substitute, as required
- Black pepper, as required
- 8 large lettuce leaves (such as butter lettuce)

Directions:

1. Inside a container, blend the cooked quinoa, cubed cucumber, cubed tomato, cubed red onion, severed parsley, lemon juice, olive oil, salt substitute, and black pepper.
2. Mix thoroughly.
3. Lay out the lettuce leaves on a flat surface.

4. Spoon the quinoa salad solution onto each lettuce leaf.

5. Fold the lettuce leaves to form cups.

6. Serve cooled.

Per serving: Calories: 150kcal; Fat: 4g; Carbs: 24gm; Protein: 5gm; Sugar: 2gm; Sodium: 20mg; Potassium: 200mg; Phosphorus: 100mg

Watermelon and Feta Skewers

Degree of Difficulty: ★☆☆☆☆

Preparation time: ten mins

Cooking time: zero mins

Servings: four

Ingredients:

- two teacups watermelon, cut into cubes
- half teacup reduced-fat feta cheese, cut into cubes
- Fresh mint leaves, for garnish

Directions:

1. Thread a watermelon cube followed by a feta cheese cube onto each skewer.

2. Replicate till the entire components are used.

3. Garnish with fresh mint leaves.

4. Serve cooled.

Per serving: Calories: 80kcal; Fat: 2g; Carbs: 14g; Protein: 4g; Sugar: 10g; Sodium: 200mg; Potassium: 200mg; Phosphorus: 80mg

Apple and Almond Butter Wraps

Degree of Difficulty: ★★★★☆

Preparation time: five mins

Cooking time: zero mins

Servings: two

Ingredients:

- two big whole wheat tortillas
- two tbsps almond butter (low-sodium, no included salt)
- one apple, thinly cut
- Ground cinnamon, as required

Directions:

1. Lay out the tortillas on a flat surface.

2. Disperse one tbsp. of almond butter on each tortilla.

3. Place apple slices on top of the almond butter.

4. Spray with ground cinnamon.

5. Roll up the tortillas tightly and cut into bite-sized pieces.

Per serving: Calories: 220kcal; Fat: 7g; Carbs: 36g; Protein: 5g; Sugar: 12g; Sodium: 20mg; Potassium: 180mg; Phosphorus: 100mg

Melon and Prosciutto Roll-Ups

Degree of Difficulty: ★★☆☆☆

Preparation time: ten mins

Cooking time: zero mins

Servings: two

Ingredients:

- four slices of prosciutto
- 8 cantaloupe or honeydew melon wedges
- Fresh basil leaves

Directions:

1. Lay out the prosciutto slices on a flat surface.
2. Place a cantaloupe or honeydew melon wedge on each prosciutto slice.
3. Top with a fresh basil leaf.
4. Roll up tightly then secure with toothpicks if needed.
5. Serve cooled.

Per serving: Calories: 160kcal; Fat: 5g; Carbs: 14g; Protein: 14g; Sugar: 12g; Sodium: 350mg; Potassium: 300mg; Phosphorus: 160mg

Caprese Skewers

Degree of Difficulty: ★☆☆☆☆

Preparation time: ten mins

Cooking time: zero mins

Servings: four

Ingredients:

- 8 cherry tomatoes
- eight small mozzarella balls
- Fresh basil leaves
- Balsamic glaze, for drizzling

Directions:

1. Thread a cherry tomato, followed by a small mozzarella ball & a fresh basil leaf, onto each skewer.
2. Replicate till the entire components are used.
3. Spray with balsamic glaze.
4. Serve cooled.

Per serving: Calories: 100kcal; Fat: 7g; Carbs: 2g; Protein: 7gm; Sugar: 1gm; Sodium: 150mg; Potassium: 100mg; Phosphorus: 80mg

Baked Zucchini Chips

Degree of Difficulty: ★★★★☆

Preparation time: fifteen mins

Cooking time: twenty-five mins

Servings: two

Ingredients:

- one medium zucchini, thinly cut
- one tbsp olive oil
- Salt substitute, as required
- Black pepper, as required

Directions:

1. Warm up the oven to 425°F.
2. Inside a container, throw the thinly cut zucchini with olive oil, salt substitute, and black pepper.
3. Bring the zucchini slices on a baking tray in a single layer.

4. Bake in your warmed up oven for 20-25 mins or till crispy & golden brown, flipping halfway through.

5. Allow to cool prior to serving.

Per serving: Calories: 80kcal; Fat: 6g; Carbs: 6g; Protein: 2gm; Sugar: 4g; Sodium: 20mg; Potassium: 350mg; Phosphorus: 50mg

Yogurt and Berry Popsicles

Degree of Difficulty: ★★☆☆☆

Preparation time: five mins

Cooking time: four hrs (freezing time)

Servings: four

Ingredients:

- one teacup plain low-fat yogurt
- half teacup mixed berries (strawberries, blueberries, raspberries)
- one tbsp honey

Directions:

1. Inside a mixer, blend the plain yogurt, mixed berries, and honey (if anticipated).

2. Mix till even.

3. Pour the solution into popsicle molds.

4. Insert popsicle sticks into each mold.

5. Freeze for almost four hrs or 'til entirely frozen.

6. Take out from the molds and serve.

Per serving: Calories: 70kcal; Fat: 1g; Carbs: 13g; Protein: 4g; Sugar: 10g; Sodium: 50mg; Potassium: 180mg; Phosphorus: 90mg

Turkey Lettuce Wraps

Degree of Difficulty: ★★★☆☆

Preparation time: fifteen mins

Cooking time: ten mins

Servings: two

Ingredients:

- 8 large lettuce leaves (such as iceberg or romaine)
- 8 ounces ground turkey
- quarter teacup cubed bell pepper
- quarter teacup cubed zucchini
- quarter teacup cubed mushrooms
- quarter teacup cubed onion
- one piece garlic, crushed
- one tbsp low-sodium soy sauce
- one tsp sesame oil
- Salt substitute, as required
- Black pepper, as required

Directions:

1. Heat your griddle across middling temp. and spray with cooking spray.

2. Include the ground turkey then cook till browned and cooked through, breaking it up into crumbles.

3. Include the cubed bell pepper, cubed zucchini, cubed mushrooms, cubed onion, & crushed garlic to the griddle.

4. Cook for an additional five mins or till the vegetables are soft.

63

5. Stir in the low-sodium soy sauce and sesame oil.

6. Flavour with salt substitute and black pepper.

7. Spoon the turkey solution in to the lettuce leaves and roll up.

8. Secure with toothpicks if needed.

9. Serve instantly.

Per serving: Calories: 200kcal; Fat: 10g; Carbs: 10g; Protein: 20g; Sugar: 4g; Sodium: 180mg; Potassium: 380mg; Phosphorus: 180mg

Zucchini and Corn Fritters

Degree of Difficulty: ★★★★☆

Preparation time: twenty mins

Cooking time: twenty mins

Servings: 4

Ingredients:

- two medium zucchinis, grated
- one teacup frozen corn kernels, thawed
- quarter teacup cubed red onion
- two pieces garlic, crushed
- quarter teacup grated Parmesan cheese
- quarter teacup whole wheat flour
- two big eggs
- two tbsps severed fresh parsley
- one tsp baking powder
- Salt substitute, as required
- Black pepper, as required
- Cooking spray

Directions:

1. Place the grated zucchini in a colander then spray with salt substitute. Let it sit for around ten mins to release excess moisture. Squeeze out any remaining liquid.

2. Inside a big container, blend the grated zucchini, thawed corn kernels, cubed red onion, crushed garlic, grated Parmesan cheese, whole wheat flour, eggs, severed parsley, baking powder, salt substitute, and black pepper. Mix thoroughly.

3. Warm a non-stick griddle in a middling temp. and spray with cooking spray.

4. Drop spoonful of the zucchini and corn solution onto the griddle, flattening them mildly with the back of the spoon.

5. Cook for around three to four mins on all sides or till golden brown and cooked through.

6. Replicate with the rest of the solution, including more cooking spray as required.

7. Take out from the griddle then drain on paper towels.

8. Serve warm.

Per serving: Calories: 140kcal; Fat: 5g; Carbs: 17g; Protein: 7gm; Sugar: 4g; Sodium: 200mg; Potassium: 300mg; Phosphorus: 120mg

Blueberry Oat Muffins

Degree of Difficulty: ★★★☆☆

Preparation time: fifteen mins

Cooking time: twenty mins

Servings: six

Ingredients:

- one teacup rolled oats
- half teacup whole wheat flour
- half tsp baking powder
- quarter tsp baking soda
- quarter tsp cinnamon
- quarter tsp salt substitute
- quarter teacup unsweetened applesauce
- quarter teacup honey
- quarter teacup low-fat milk
- one big egg
- half tsp vanilla extract
- half teacup fresh blueberries

Directions:

1. Warm up the oven to 375°F. Cover a muffin tin with paper liners or oil the tin.
2. In your medium container, blend the rolled oats, whole wheat flour, cinnamon, baking powder, baking soda, and salt substitute.
3. Inside another container, whisk collectively the unsweetened applesauce, honey, low-fat milk, egg, and vanilla extract.
4. Bring the wet components into the dry components and stir till just blended.
5. Gently fold in the fresh blueberries.
6. Place the batter equally between the muffin cups.
7. Bake in your warmed up oven for 18-20 mins or 'til a toothpick introduced into the middle comes out clean.
8. Let the muffins to cool in the tin for a couple of mins prior to placing them to a wire rack to cool entirely.

Per serving: Calories: 150kcal; Fat: 2g; Carbs: 30g; Protein: 4g; Sugar: 15g; Sodium: 120mg; Potassium: 180mg; Phosphorus: 120mg

Spinach and Feta Stuffed Mushrooms

Degree of Difficulty: ★★★★☆

Preparation time: fifteen mins

Cooking time: twenty mins

Servings: two

Ingredients:

- 8 large button mushrooms
- two teacups fresh spinach leaves
- quarter teacup crumbled feta cheese
- two tbsps cubed red onion
- one piece garlic, crushed
- one tsp olive oil
- Salt substitute, as required
- Black pepper, as required

Directions:

1. Warm up the oven to 375°F.

2. Take out the stems from the mushrooms then put away.

3. Inside your griddle, warm the olive oil in a middling temp.

4. Include the crushed garlic then cubed red onion to the griddle and cook till fragrant.

5. Include the spinach leaves then cook till wilted.

6. Take out from heat and let cool mildly.

7. Chop the mushroom stems then include them to the griddle along with the crumbled feta cheese.

8. Flavour with salt substitute and black pepper.

9. Spoon the spinach and feta solution into the mushroom caps.

10. Bring the stuffed mushrooms on a baking tray.

11. Bake in your warmed up oven for 15-20 mins or till the mushrooms are soft.

12. Allow to cool mildly prior to serving.

Per serving: Calories: 140kcal; Fat: 8g; Carbs: 11g; Protein: 9g; Sugar: 3g; Sodium: 180mg; Potassium: 300mg; Phosphorus: 200mg

Baked Eggplant Chips

Degree of Difficulty: ★★★☆

Preparation time: fifteen mins

Cooking time: twenty mins

Servings: 2

Ingredients:

- one small eggplant
- one tbsp olive oil
- Salt substitute, as required
- Black pepper, as required
- quarter teacup grated Parmesan cheese

Directions:

1. Warm up the oven to 425°F.

2. Slice the eggplant into thin rounds.

3. Inside a container, throw the eggplant slices with olive oil, salt substitute, and black pepper.

4. Organize the seasoned eggplant slices on a baking tray inside a single layer.

5. Spray grated Parmesan cheese uniformly over the eggplant slices.

6. Bake in your warmed up oven for fifteen to twenty mins or till golden brown and crispy.

7. Allow to cool prior to serving.

Per serving: Calories: 120kcal; Fat: 7g; Carbs: 10g; Protein: 4g; Sugar: 4g; Sodium: 100mg; Potassium: 250mg; Phosphorus: 100mg

Cucumber Roll-Ups

Degree of Difficulty: ★★☆☆

Preparation time: ten mins

Cooking time: zero mins

Servings: two

Ingredients:

- one big cucumber
- 4 slices of low-sodium deli turkey or chicken
- 4 slices of low-sodium Swiss cheese
- Mustard or low-sodium mayonnaise (optional)

Directions:

1. Slice the cucumber lengthwise into fine strips utilizing a vegetable peeler or a mandoline.
2. Lay out a cucumber strip and place a slice of turkey or chicken and a slice of Swiss cheese on top.
3. Roll up tightly then secure with toothpicks if needed.
4. Replicate with the rest of the cucumber strips and filling components.
5. Optional: Disperse a thin layer of mustard or low-sodium mayonnaise on the cucumber strip prior to including the turkey or chicken and cheese.
6. Serve cooled.

Per serving: Calories: 120kcal; Fat: 5g; Carbs: 5gm; Protein: 14g; Sugar: 3g; Sodium: 150mg; Potassium: 300mg; Phosphorus: 200mg

Carrot and Ginger Soup

Degree of Difficulty: ★★★☆☆

Preparation time: fifteen mins

Cooking time: thirty mins

Servings: 2

Ingredients:

- 4 large carrots, skinned and cubed
- one small onion, severed
- 1" piece of fresh ginger, skinned & grated
- 3 teacups low-sodium vegetable broth
- one tbsp olive oil
- Salt substitute, as required
- Black pepper, as required
- Fresh cilantro, for garnish (optional)

Directions:

1. Warm the olive oil in your huge pot across middling temp..
2. Include the severed onion and grated ginger to the pot and cook till the onion is soft and luminous.
3. Place the cubed carrots to the pot and cook for a couple of mins.
4. Pour in the low-sodium vegetable broth and raise to a boil.
5. Lower the heat then simmer for around twenty-thirty mins or till the carrots are soft.
6. Take out from heat and let cool mildly.
7. Utilize an immersion mixer or bring the solution to a mixer then blend till even.
8. Flavour with salt substitute and black pepper.
9. Garnish with fresh cilantro if anticipated.
10. Serve warm.

Per serving: Calories: 120kcal; Fat: 4g; Sodium: 150mg; Potassium: 300mg; Carbs: 20g; Protein: 2gm; Sugar: 10g; Phosphorus: 60mg

Dessert Recipes

Watermelon Granita

Degree of Difficulty: ★★☆☆☆

Preparation time: ten mins (plus freezing time)

Cooking time: N/A

Servings: four

Ingredients:

- four teacups cubed seedless watermelon
- two tbsps fresh lime juice
- two tbsps honey or sugar (optional)

Directions:

1. Place the watermelon cubes inside a mixer then blend till even.
2. Include lime juice and sweeten with honey or sugar if anticipated.
3. Bring the solution into a shallow dish and put in the freezer.
4. Every thirty mins, scrape the solution using a fork to create a granita texture.
5. Replicate the scraping process for around 2 hours or till the granita is fully frozen.
6. Serve in cooled bowls.

Per serving: Calories: 50kcal; Fat: 0.5g; Carbs: 13g; Protein: 1g; Sugar: 10g; Sodium: 0mg; Potassium: 150mg; Phosphorus: 20mg

Orange Sherbet

Degree of Difficulty: ★★★☆☆

Preparation time: five mins (plus freezing time)

Cooking time: N/A

Servings: 4

Ingredients:

- two teacups freshly squeezed orange juice
- one tbsp honey or sugar

Directions:

1. Inside your container, blend the orange juice and honey or sugar.
2. Stir till the sweetener is dissolved.
3. Bring the solution into a shallow dish and place in the freezer.
4. Every 30 mins, scrape the solution with a fork to break up the ice crystals.
5. Replicate the scraping process for around 2 hours or till the sherbet is fully frozen.
6. Serve in cooled bowls.

Per serving: Calories: 60kcal; Fat: 0.5g; Carbs: 15g; Protein: 1g; Sugar: 11g; Sodium: 0mg; Potassium: 250mg; Phosphorus: 15mg

Pears with Honey and Cinnamon

Degree of Difficulty: ★★☆☆☆

Preparation time: ten mins

Cooking time: fifteen mins

Servings: 2

Ingredients:

- two ripe pears, halved and cored
- two tbsps honey
- half tsp ground cinnamon

Directions:

1. Warm up the oven to 375°F.
2. Put the pear halves, cut side up, in a baking tray.
3. Spray honey over each pear half and spray with ground cinnamon.
4. Bake for around fifteen mins or till the pears are soft.
5. Serve warm.

Per serving: Calories: 120kcal; Fat: 0.5g; Carbs: 32g; Protein: 0.5g; Sugar: 26g; Sodium: 0mg; Potassium: 200mg; Phosphorus: 10mg

Baked Apples with Cinnamon

Degree of Difficulty: ★★☆☆

Preparation time: ten mins

Cooking time: twenty-five mins

Servings: 2

Ingredients:

- two medium-sized apples (Granny Smith or any firm variety)
- one tbsp unsalted butter, dissolved
- one tbsp brown sugar
- half tsp ground cinnamon

Directions:

1. Warm up the oven to 375°F.
2. Core the apples and cut off the top third.
3. Inside your small container, mix dissolved butter, brown sugar, and cinnamon.
4. Brush the apples with the solution, ensuring to cover the inside.
5. Put the apples in a baking tray and bake for around twenty-five mins or 'til soft.
6. Serve warm.

Per serving: Calories: 130kcal; Fat: 4gm; Carbs: 25g; Protein: 0.5g; Sugar: 19g; Sodium: 0mg; Potassium: 190mg; Phosphorus: 15mg

Strawberry Frozen Yogurt

Degree of Difficulty: ★★★☆

Preparation time: ten mins (plus freezing time)

Cooking time: N/A

Servings: four

Ingredients:

- two teacups frozen strawberries
- one teacup plain Greek yogurt
- two tbsps honey or sugar (optional)

Directions:

1. Inside your mixer or mixing container, blend frozen strawberries, Greek yogurt, and honey or sugar.
2. Blend till even and creamy.

3. Taste and adjust the sweetness if anticipated.

4. Transfer the solution to a freezer-safe container and freeze for around three-four hrs or till firm.

5. Allow the frozen yogurt to soften for a couple of mins prior to serving.

Per serving: Calories: 80kcal; Fat: 0.5g; Carbs: 16g; Protein: 6g; Sugar: 11g; Sodium: 25mg; Potassium: 200mg; Phosphorus: 70mg

Pineapple Coconut Smoothie

Degree of Difficulty: ★★☆☆☆

Preparation time: five mins

Cooking time: N/A

Servings: 2

Ingredients:

- two teacups cubed fresh pineapple
- one teacup unsweetened coconut milk
- half teacup plain Greek yogurt
- two tbsps honey or sugar (optional)
- Ice cubes (optional)

Directions:

1. Inside a mixer, blend cubed pineapple, coconut milk, Greek yogurt, and honey or sugar.

2. Blend till even and creamy.

3. Place ice cubes if anticipated and blend again till well incorporated.

4. Serve cooled.

Per serving: Calories: 150kcal; Fat: 5g; Carbs: 26gm; Protein: 5gm; Sugar: 19g; Sodium: 35mg; Potassium: 230mg; Phosphorus: 120mg

Raspberry Chia Jam

Degree of Difficulty: ★★★☆☆

Preparation time: five mins (plus chilling time)

Cooking time: N/A

Servings: 8

Ingredients:

- two teacups fresh raspberries
- two tbsps chia seeds
- two tbsps honey or sugar (optional)
- half tsp lemon juice

Directions:

1. Inside a container, mash the raspberries with a fork.

2. Include chia seeds, honey or sugar, and lemon juice.

3. Stir thoroughly to blend.

4. Cover your container then put in the fridge for almost 1 hour or till the solution denses and resembles jam.

5. Stir again prior to serving.

6. Place inside a sealed container in your fridge for almost a week.

Per serving: Calories: 30kcal; Fat: 1g; Carbs: 5g; Protein: 1g; Sugar: 3g; Sodium: 0mg; Potassium: 60mg; Phosphorus: 20mg

Apple Cinnamon Muffins

Degree of Difficulty: ★★★☆☆

Preparation time: fifteen mins

Cooking time: twenty mins

Servings: 12

Ingredients:

- one and half teacups all-purpose flour
- half teacup oat flour
- half teacup granulated sugar
- two tsps baking powder
- one tsp ground cinnamon
- quarter tsp salt
- one teacup unsweetened applesauce
- quarter teacup vegetable oil
- quarter teacup unsweetened almond milk
- one tsp vanilla extract
- one big apple, skinned and cubed

Directions:

1. Warm up the oven to 375 deg. F and cover a muffin tin with paper liners.
2. Inside a big container, whisk collectively all-purpose flour, oat flour, cinnamon, sugar, baking powder and salt.
3. Inside a separate container, blend applesauce, vegetable oil, almond milk, and vanilla extract.
4. Bring the wet components into the dry components and mix till just blended.
5. Gently fold in the cubed apple.
6. Split the batter equally between all muffin cups, filling all about 2/3 full.
7. Bake for approximately twenty mins or 'til a toothpick introduced into the middle comes out clean.
8. Let the muffins to cool in the tin for a couple of mins prior to bringing to a wire rack to cool entirely.

Per serving: Calories: 150kcal; Fat: 5g; Carbs: 25g; Protein: 3g; Sugar: 10g; Sodium: 100mg; Potassium: 80mg; Phosphorus: 70mg

Blueberry Oat Bars

Degree of Difficulty: ★★★☆☆

Preparation time: fifteen mins

Cooking time: thirty mins

Servings: 9

Ingredients:

- one teacup old-fashioned rolled oats
- half teacup all-purpose flour
- quarter teacup packed brown sugar
- quarter tsp baking soda
- quarter tsp salt
- quarter teacup unsalted butter, dissolved
- quarter teacup unsweetened applesauce
- quarter teacup honey or sugar
- half tsp vanilla extract
- one teacup fresh blueberries

Directions:

1. Warm up your oven to 350 deg. F then cover an 8x8-inch baking tray with parchment paper.
2. Inside a big container, blend oats, flour, brown sugar, baking soda, and salt.
3. Inside a separate container, mix dissolved butter, applesauce, honey or sugar, and vanilla extract.
4. Place the wet components to the dry components and mix till thoroughly blended.
5. Gently fold in the blueberries.
6. Press the solution uniformly in to the prepared baking tray.
7. Bake for around twenty-five to thirty mins or till golden brown.
8. Let the bars to cool entirely prior to cutting into squares.

Per serving: Calories: 160kcal; Fat: 6g; Carbs: 25g; Protein: 3g; Sugar: 12g; Sodium: 80mg; Potassium: 70mg; Phosphorus: 55mg

Baked Peaches with Cinnamon

Degree of Difficulty: ★★☆☆☆

Preparation time: ten mins

Cooking time: fifteen mins

Servings: two

Ingredients:

- two ripe peaches
- one tbsp unsalted butter, dissolved
- one tbsp brown sugar
- half tsp ground cinnamon

Directions:

1. Warm up the oven to 375°F.
2. Cut the peaches in half and take out the pits.
3. Place the peach halves, cut side up, in a baking tray.
4. Inside your small container, mix dissolved butter, brown sugar, and cinnamon.
5. Brush the solution over the peaches.
6. Bake for around fifteen mins or till the peaches are soft.
7. Serve warm.

Per serving: Calories: 90kcal; Fat: 3.5g; Carbs: 15g; Protein: 1g; Sugar: 13gm; Sodium: 0mg; Potassium: 250mg; Phosphorus: 15mg

Coconut Rice Pudding

Degree of Difficulty: ★★★☆☆

Preparation time: five mins

Cooking time: forty-five mins

Servings: four

Ingredients:

- one teacup cooked white rice
- one tin (13.5 oz) light coconut milk
- two tbsps honey or sugar
- half tsp vanilla extract
- quarter tsp ground cinnamon
- quarter teacup unsweetened shredded coconut, toasted

Directions:

1. Inside a medium-sized saucepan, blend cooked rice, coconut milk, honey or sugar, vanilla extract, and ground cinnamon.

2. Cook in a middling temp., mixing irregularly, for around thirty-forty mins or till the solution denses to a pudding consistency.

3. Take out from heat then let it cool midly.

4. Serve warm or cooled, spray with toasted shredded coconut if anticipated.

Per serving: Calories: 220kcal; Fat: 9g; Carbs: 33g; Protein: 3g; Sugar: 12g; Sodium: 20mg; Potassium: 160mg; Phosphorus: 70mg

Vanilla Rice Pudding

Degree of Difficulty: ★★★☆☆

Preparation time: five mins

Cooking time: thirty mins

Servings: four

Ingredients:

- half teacup Arborio rice
- two teacups unsweetened almond milk
- two tbsps honey or sugar
- half tsp vanilla extract
- Ground cinnamon for garnish

Directions:

1. Inside a medium-sized saucepan, blend Arborio rice, almond milk, honey or sugar, and vanilla extract.

2. Raise the solution to a boil in a middling temp., stirring frequently.

3. Decrease the temp. to low and simmer for around twenty-thirty mins, mixing irregularly, till the rice is cooked and the pudding denses.

4. Take out from heat then let it cool mildly.

5. Spray with ground cinnamon prior to serving.

6. Serve warm or cooled.

Per serving: Calories: 170kcal; Fat: 2.5g; Carbs: 33g; Protein: 3g; Sugar: 12g; Sodium: 85mg; Potassium: 90mg; Phosphorus: 90mg

Carrot Cake Muffins

Degree of Difficulty: ★★★☆☆

Preparation time: fifteen mins

Cooking time: twenty mins

Servings: twelve

Ingredients:

- one and half teacups all-purpose flour
- half teacup rolled oats
- half teacup packed brown sugar
- one tsp baking powder
- half tsp baking soda
- half tsp ground cinnamon
- quarter tsp ground nutmeg
- quarter tsp salt
- half teacup unsweetened applesauce
- quarter teacup vegetable oil
- two eggs

74

- one tsp vanilla extract
- one teacup grated carrots
- quarter teacup severed walnuts (optional)

Directions:

1. Warm up the oven to 375 deg. F and cover a muffin tin with paper liners.

2. Inside a big container, whisk collectively flour, oats, brown sugar, cinnamon, baking powder, baking soda, nutmeg, and salt.

3. Inside a separate container, blend applesauce, vegetable oil, eggs, and vanilla extract.

4. Bring the wet components into the dry components and mix till just blended.

5. Gently fold in grated carrots and severed walnuts (if using).

6. Split the batter uniformly between all muffin teacups, filling each around 2/3 full.

7. Bake for approximately eighteen-twenty mins or 'til a toothpick introduced in the middle comes out clean.

8. Let the muffins to cool in the tin for a couple of mins prior to bringing to a wire rack to cool entirely.

Per serving: Calories: 160kcal; Fat: 6g; Carbs: 24g; Protein: 4g; Sugar: 11g; Sodium: 110mg; Potassium: 80mg; Phosphorus: 55mg

Lemon Poppy Seed Muffins

Degree of Difficulty: ★★★☆☆

Preparation time: fifteen mins

Cooking time: twenty mins

Servings: 12

Ingredients:

- one and half teacups all-purpose flour
- half teacup granulated sugar
- one tbsp poppy seeds
- one tbsp lemon zest
- two tsps baking powder
- quarter tsp salt
- half teacup unsweetened almond milk
- quarter teacup vegetable oil
- quarter teacup fresh lemon juice
- half tsp vanilla extract

Directions:

1. Warm up the oven to 375 deg. F and cover a muffin tin with paper liners.

2. Inside a big container, whisk collectively flour, sugar, poppy seeds, lemon zest, baking powder, and salt.

3. Inside a separate container, blend almond milk, vegetable oil, lemon juice, and vanilla extract.

4. Bring the wet components into the dry components then mix 'til just blended.

5. Split the batter equally among all muffin cups, filling each around 2/3 full.

6. Bake for approximately eighteen-twenty mins or 'til a toothpick injected in the middle comes out clean.

7. Let the muffins to cool in the tin for a couple of mins prior to bringing to a wire rack to cool entirely.

Per serving: Calories: 150kcal; Fat: 5g; Carbs: 24gm; Protein: 3gm; Sugar: 10g; Sodium: 100mg; Potassium: 60mg; Phosphorus: 70mg

Peach Crumble

Degree of Difficulty: ★★★☆☆

Preparation time: fifteen mins

Cooking time: twenty-five mins

Servings: 4

Ingredients:

- 4 medium-sized peaches, skinned and cut
- one tbsp lemon juice
- two tbsps honey or sugar
- half tsp ground cinnamon
- half teacup rolled oats
- quarter teacup all-purpose flour
- two tbsps unsalted butter, dissolved
- two tbsps severed almonds (optional)

Directions:

1. Warm up the oven to 375°F.
2. Inside your container, throw the cut peaches with lemon juice, honey or sugar, and cinnamon.
3. Raise the peach solution to a baking tray.
4. Inside your separate container, blend rolled oats, flour, dissolved butter, and severed almonds (if using).

5. Spray the oat solution uniformly in the peaches.
6. Bake for around twenty-five mins or till the crumble is golden brown and the peaches are soft.
7. Serve warm or at room temp.

Per serving: Calories: 180kcal; Fat: 6g; Carbs: 31g; Protein: 4g; Sugar: 19g; Sodium: 0mg; Potassium: 290mg; Phosphorus: 65mg

Honeydew Lime Sorbet

Degree of Difficulty: ★★★★☆

Preparation time: ten mins (plus freezing time)

Cooking time: N/A

Servings: four

Ingredients:

- four teacups cubed honeydew melon
- two tbsps fresh lime juice
- two tbsps honey or sugar
- Fresh mint leaves for garnish

Directions:

1. Place the cubed honeydew melon inside a mixer and blend till even.
2. Include lime juice and sweeten with honey or sugar if anticipated.
3. Bring the solution into a shallow dish and put in the freezer.
4. Every 30 mins, scrape the solution with a fork to create a sorbet texture.

5. Replicate the scraping process for around 2 hours or till the sorbet is fully frozen.

6. Serve in cooled bowls then garnish with fresh mint leaves if anticipated.

Per serving: Calories: 60kcal; Fat: 0.5g; Carbs: 16g; Protein: 1g; Sugar: 15g; Sodium: 15mg; Potassium: 230mg; Phosphorus: 20mg

Chocolate Mousse

Degree of Difficulty: ★★★☆☆
Preparation time: five mins
Cooking time: five mins
Servings: two
Ingredients:

- quarter teacup unsweetened cocoa powder
- quarter tsp vanilla
- three-quarter teacup heavy cream
- two oz cream cheese
- 4 drops liquid stevia

Directions:

1. Put the entire components into the mixer then blend till even and creamy.

2. Pour solution into the serving containers and put in the fridge for 1-2 hours.

3. Serve and relish.

Per serving: Calories: 255kcal; Fat: 24g; Carbs: 6g; Protein: 5.1g; Sugar: 12g; Sodium: 75mg; Potassium: 117mg; Phosphorus: 110mg

Mango Yogurt Parfait

Degree of Difficulty: ★★☆☆☆

Preparation time: ten mins
Cooking time: N/A
Servings: one
Ingredients:

- half teacup cubed mango
- half teacup plain Greek yogurt
- two tbsps low-sugar granola
- one tbsp severed almonds

Directions:

1. In a glass or container, layer the cubed mango, Greek yogurt, and granola.

2. Replicate the layers till the entire components are utilized.

3. Spray severed almonds on top if anticipated.

4. Serve instantly.

Per serving: Calories: 220kcal; Fat: 5gm; Carbs: 35g; Protein: 10g; Sugar: 25g; Sodium: 60mg; Potassium: 300mg; Phosphorus: 150mg

Cinnamon Rice Cakes

Degree of Difficulty: ★★★☆☆
Preparation time: ten mins
Cooking time: twenty mins
Servings: four
Ingredients:

- two teacups cooked white rice
- two tbsps unsalted butter, dissolved
- two tbsps honey or sugar

- one tsp ground cinnamon
- quarter tsp vanilla extract

Directions:

1. Inside a big container, blend cooked rice, dissolved butter, honey or sugar, ground cinnamon, and vanilla extract.

2. Mix thoroughly till the entire components are uniformly combined.

3. Shape the solution into small patties or balls.

4. Heat your non-stick griddle across middling temp. and mildly oil it with cooking spray.

5. Cook the rice cakes for around three to four mins on all sides or till golden brown and crispy.

6. Serve warm.

Per serving: Calories: 180kcal; Fat: 6g; Carbs: 30g; Protein: 2gm; Sugar: 11g; Sodium: 5mg; Potassium: 50mg; Phosphorus: 50mg

Lemon Yogurt Cake

Degree of Difficulty: ★★★☆☆
Preparation time: fifteen mins
Cooking time: forty-five mins
Servings: eight
Ingredients:

- one and half teacups all-purpose flour
- one tsp baking powder
- quarter tsp baking soda
- quarter tsp salt
- half teacup unsalted butter, softened
- one teacup granulated sugar
- two eggs
- half teacup plain Greek yogurt
- quarter teacup fresh lemon juice
- two tbsps lemon zest
- half tsp vanilla extract
- Powdered sugar for dusting (optional)

Directions:

1. Warm up your oven to 350 deg. F then oil a 9x5-inch loaf pot.

2. Inside a medium-sized container, whisk collectively flour, baking powder, baking soda, and salt.

3. Inside your separate big container, cream collectively butter and sugar till light and fluffy.

4. Whisk in the eggs, one at a time, followed by the lemon juice, lemon zest, and vanilla extract.

5. Slowly place the flour solution to the wet components, mixing till just blend.

6. Fold in the Greek yogurt till the batter is even.

7. Bring the batter into the prepared loaf pan then even the top.

8. Bake for almost forty to forty-five mins or 'til a toothpick introduced in the middle comes out clean.

9. Let the cake to cool in your pot for ten mins, then bring it to a wire rack to cool entirely.

10. Pour with powdered sugar prior to serving, if anticipated.

Per serving: Calories: 290kcal; Fat: 12g; Carbs: 40g; Protein: 5g; Sugar: 24g; Sodium: 150mg; Potassium: 90mg; Phosphorus: 110mg

Special Recipes

Baked Cod with Herbs

Degree of Difficulty: ★★☆☆☆

Preparation time: ten mins

Cooking time: twenty mins

Servings: 2

Ingredients:

- two cod fillets
- one tbsp olive oil
- one tbsp fresh parsley, severed
- one tbsp fresh thyme, severed
- one tsp lemon zest
- Salt and pepper as required

Directions:

1. Warm up the oven to 400°F.
2. Bring the cod fillets in a baking tray and spray with olive oil.
3. Spray the fresh parsley, fresh thyme, lemon zest, salt, and pepper over the fish.
4. Bake for fifteen-twenty mins or till the cod flakes simply with a fork.
5. Serve warm.

Per serving: Calories: 200kcal; Fat: 7g; Carbs: 1g; Protein: 35g; Sugar: 0g; Sodium: 90mg; Potassium: 360mg; Phosphorus: 280mg

Vegetable Stir-Fry

Degree of Difficulty: ★★☆☆☆

Preparation time: ten mins

Cooking time: ten mins

Servings: four

Ingredients:

- one tbsp olive oil
- one onion, cut
- two pieces of garlic, crushed
- 1 carrot, julienned
- one bell pepper, cut
- one zucchini, cut
- one teacup broccoli florets
- two tbsps low-sodium soy sauce
- one tbsp rice vinegar
- half tsp ginger, grated
- half tsp sesame oil

Directions:

1. Warm the olive oil in a huge griddle or wok at medium-high temp.
2. Include the cut onion and crushed garlic. Cook for two-three mins till softened.
3. Include the julienned carrot, cut bell pepper, cut zucchini, and broccoli florets to the griddle. Stir-fry for around five to six mins or till the vegetables are soft-crisp.

4. Inside a small container, whisk collectively the low-sodium soy sauce, rice vinegar, ginger, and sesame oil.

5. Pour the sauce over the stir-fried vegetables and cook for another min, blending thoroughly.

6. Serve warm.

Per serving: Calories: 120kcal; Fat: 5gm; Carbs: 14g; Protein: 5g; Sugar: 6g; Sodium: 210mg; Potassium: 300mg; Phosphorus: 90mg

Baked White Fish with Herbs

Degree of Difficulty: ★★☆☆☆

Preparation time: ten mins

Cooking time: twenty mins

Servings: two

Ingredients:

- 2 white fish fillets (like tilapia or sole)
- one tbsp olive oil
- one tbsp fresh dill, severed
- one tbsp fresh parsley, severed
- one tsp lemon zest
- Salt and pepper as required

Directions:

1. Warm up the oven to 400°F.

2. Bring the white fish fillets in a baking tray. Spray with olive oil then spray with fresh dill, fresh parsley, lemon zest, salt, and pepper.

3. Bake for fifteen-twenty mins or till the fish flakes simply with a fork.

4. Serve warm.

Per serving: Calories: 180kcal; Fat: 6g; Carbs: 0g; Protein: 30g; Sugar: 0g; Sodium: 70mg; Potassium: 280mg; Phosphorus: 270mg

Grilled Salmon with Dill Sauce

Degree of Difficulty: ★★☆☆☆

Preparation time: ten mins

Cooking time: fifteen mins

Servings: two

Ingredients:

- two salmon fillets
- one tbsp olive oil
- one tbsp fresh dill, severed
- one tbsp lemon juice
- Salt and pepper as required

Directions:

1. Warm up the grill to medium-high temp.

2. Rub the salmon fillets using olive oil and flavour with salt and pepper.

3. Grill the salmon for around six-eight mins on all sides or till cooked through.

4. Inside a small container, blend collectively the fresh dill and lemon juice.

5. Serve the grilled salmon with the dill sauce on top.

Per serving: Calories: 300kcal; Fat: 18g; Carbs: 1g; Protein: 34g; Sugar: 0g; Sodium:

80mg; Potassium: 320mg; Phosphorus: 240mg

Roasted Vegetable Medley

Degree of Difficulty: ★★☆☆☆

Preparation time: fifteen mins

Cooking time: thirty mins

Servings: four

Ingredients:

- 1 sweet potato, skinned and cubed
- two carrots, skinned and cut
- one zucchini, cut
- one red onion, cut into wedges
- one bell pepper, cut
- one tbsp olive oil
- one tsp dried thyme
- one tsp dried rosemary
- Salt and pepper as required

Directions:

1. Warm up the oven to 425°F.
2. Inside a big container, throw together the cubed sweet potato, cut carrots, cut zucchini, red onion wedges, and cut bell pepper with olive oil, dried thyme, dried rosemary, salt, and pepper.
3. Disperse the vegetables in a one layer onto a baking tray.
4. Roast in the oven for twenty-five to thirty mins or till the vegetables are soft and mildly caramelized, stirring halfway through.

5. Serve warm.

Per serving: Calories: 150kcal; Fat: 4g; Carbs: 28g; Protein: 3gm; Sugar: 7g; Sodium: 60mg; Potassium: 300mg; Phosphorus: 80mg

Turkey and Vegetable Skewers

Degree of Difficulty: ★★★★☆

Preparation time: fifteen mins

Cooking time: ten mins

Servings: four

Ingredients:

- one lb. turkey breast, cut into 1" cubes
- one red bell pepper, that is cut into 1" pieces
- one zucchini, cut into half inch rounds
- one red onion, cut into 1" pieces
- two tbsps olive oil
- one tsp dried oregano
- half tsp garlic powder
- Salt and pepper as required

Directions:

1. Warm up the grill or broiler.
2. Thread the turkey cubes, red bell pepper pieces, zucchini rounds, and red onion pieces onto skewers.
3. Inside your small container, blend the olive oil, dried oregano, garlic powder, salt, and pepper. Brush the solution over the skewered turkey and vegetables.

4. Grill or broil the skewers for around four to five mins on all sides or till the turkey is cooked through and the vegetables are soft.

5. Serve warm.

Per serving: Calories: 180kcal; Fat: 6g; Carbs: 6g; Protein: 25g; Sugar: 3g; Sodium: 90mg; Potassium: 380mg; Phosphorus: 220mg

Roasted Cauliflower and Chickpea Salad

Degree of Difficulty: ★★☆☆☆

Preparation time: fifteen mins

Cooking time: twenty-five mins

Servings: 4

Ingredients:

- 1 head cauliflower, cut into florets
- one tin chickpeas, drained and washed
- two tbsps olive oil
- one tsp ground cumin
- half tsp paprika
- Salt and pepper as required
- four teacups mixed salad greens
- quarter teacup severed fresh parsley
- quarter teacup severed fresh mint
- two tbsps lemon juice
- two tbsps olive oil
- Salt and pepper as required

Directions:

1. Warm up the oven to 425°F.

2. Inside a big container, throw together the cauliflower florets, drained and washed chickpeas, olive oil, ground cumin, paprika, salt, and pepper till well covered.

3. Disperse the cauliflower and chickpea solution in a lone layer on a baking tray.

4. Roast in the oven for twenty to twenty-five mins or till the cauliflower is soft and golden brown, stirring halfway through.

5. Inside a separate container, blend the mixed salad greens, severed fresh parsley, severed fresh mint, lemon juice, olive oil, salt, and pepper. Throw well to blend.

6. Serve the roasted cauliflower and chickpeas on top of the mixed salad greens.

Per serving: Calories: 240kcal; Fat: 12g; Carbs: 28g; Protein: 8g; Sugar: 4g; Sodium: 180mg; Potassium: 320mg; Phosphorus: 160mg

Shrimp and Broccoli Stir-Fry

Degree of Difficulty: ★★☆☆☆

Preparation time: ten mins

Cooking time: ten mins

Servings: 2

Ingredients:

- 8 oz. shrimp, skinned and deveined
- one tbsp olive oil
- two pieces of garlic, crushed
- one tsp ginger, grated
- two teacups broccoli florets

- one red bell pepper, cut
- two tbsps low-sodium soy sauce
- one tbsp rice vinegar
- half tsp sesame oil
- one tbsp sesame seeds (optional)

Directions:

1. Warm the olive oil in a huge griddle or wok at medium-high temp..
2. Include the crushed garlic and grated ginger. Cook for one min till fragrant.
3. Place the shrimp to the griddle and cook for two-three mins 'til pink and cooked through. Take the shrimp from the griddle and put away.
4. Inside your identical griddle, include the broccoli florets and cut red bell pepper. Stir-fry for around four to five mins till the vegetables are soft-crisp.
5. Inside a small container, whisk collectively the low-sodium soy sauce, rice vinegar, and sesame oil.
6. Return the cooked shrimp to the griddle and pour the sauce over the shrimp & vegetables. Cook for another min, stirring well to cover all.
7. Spray with sesame seeds (optional) and serve hot.

Per serving: Calories: 220kcal; Fat: 10gm; Carbs: 12g; Protein: 20g; Sugar: 4g; Sodium: 220mg; Potassium: 300mg; Phosphorus: 240mg

Stuffed Bell Peppers

Degree of Difficulty: ★★★☆☆

Preparation time: twenty mins

Cooking time: forty mins

Servings: four

Ingredients:

- 4 bell peppers (any color), tops removed and seeds removed
- one teacup cooked brown rice
- half lb. lean ground turkey or chicken
- half onion, cubed
- two pieces of garlic, crushed
- half teacup cubed tomatoes
- quarter teacup low-sodium chicken broth
- one tsp dried oregano
- half tsp dried basil
- Salt and pepper as required

Directions:

1. Warm up the oven to 375°F.
2. Inside a huge pot of boiling water, blanch the bell peppers for five mins. Take out them from the water and put away.
3. Inside a griddle, cook the ground turkey or chicken across middling temp. till browned. Include the cubed onion & crushed garlic and cook till the onion is luminous.
4. Stir in the cooked brown rice, cubed tomatoes, low-sodium chicken broth, dried oregano, dried basil, salt, and pepper. Cook

for an additional two-three mins 'til warmed over.

5. Stuff the bell peppers with the turkey or chicken solution and place them in a baking tray.

6. Bake for thirty to thirty-five mins or 'til the peppers are soft and the filling is hot.

7. Serve warm.

Per serving: Calories: 250kcal; Fat: 6g; Carbs: 31g; Protein: 20gm; Sugar: 7g; Sodium: 120mg; Potassium: 280mg; Phosphorus: 260mg

Quinoa and Vegetable Salad

Degree of Difficulty: ★★☆☆☆

Preparation time: fifteen mins

Cooking time: fifteen mins

Servings: four

Ingredients:

- one teacup quinoa, cooked and cooled
- 1 cucumber, cubed
- one red bell pepper, cubed
- one carrot, grated
- quarter teacup fresh parsley, severed
- quarter teacup fresh mint, severed
- two tbsps lemon juice
- one tbsp olive oil
- Salt and pepper as required

Directions:

1. Inside a big container, blend the cooked and cooled quinoa, cubed cucumber, cubed red bell pepper, grated carrot, severed fresh parsley, and severed fresh mint.

2. Inside your small container, whisk collectively the lemon juice, olive oil, salt, and pepper.

3. Transfer the dressing across the quinoa and vegetables. Throw well to blend.

4. Serve cooled or at room temp.

Per serving: Calories: 180kcal; Fat: 5g; Carbs: 29g; Protein: 5g; Sugar: 4g; Sodium: 50mg; Potassium: 350mg; Phosphorus: 150mg

Roasted Chicken and Vegetables

Degree of Difficulty: ★★☆☆☆

Preparation time: fifteen mins

Cooking time: forty-five mins

Servings: four

Ingredients:

- four chicken thighs, bone-in and skin-on
- one tbsp olive oil
- one tsp dried thyme
- one tsp dried rosemary
- half tsp garlic powder
- Salt and pepper as required
- two teacups mixed vegetables (e.g., carrots, green beans, cauliflower), severed

Directions:

1. Warm up the oven to 400°F.

2. Bring the chicken thighs in a baking tray. Pour with olive oil then spray with dried

thyme, dried rosemary, salt, garlic powder, and pepper.

3. Arrange the severed mixed vegetables around the chicken thighs.

4. Roast in the oven for 40-forty-five mins or till the chicken is cooked through and the vegetables are soft.

5. Serve warm.

Per serving: Calories: 280kcal; Fat: 16g; Carbs: 10g; Protein: 23g; Sugar: 3g; Sodium: 120mg; Potassium: 380mg; Phosphorus: 230mg

Tofu Stir-Fry

Degree of Difficulty: ★★☆☆☆

Preparation time: fifteen mins

Cooking time: fifteen mins

Servings: four

Ingredients:

- one package extra-firm tofu, drained then cut into cubes
- two tbsps low-sodium soy sauce
- one tbsp rice vinegar
- one tsp sesame oil
- one tbsp olive oil
- two pieces of garlic, crushed
- one tsp ginger, grated
- one teacup cut mushrooms
- one bell pepper, cut
- one teacup snow peas
- one teacup broccoli florets

- Salt and pepper as required

Directions:

1. Inside a container, blend the tofu cubes, low-sodium soy sauce, rice vinegar, and sesame oil. Toss gently to cover the tofu uniformly. Let it marinate for ten mins.

2. Warm the olive oil inside a huge griddle or wok at medium-high temp. Include the crushed garlic and grated ginger. Cook for one min till fragrant.

3. Include the marinated tofu cubes to the griddle and cook for around three to four mins 'til browned. Take out the tofu from the griddle then put away.

4. Inside your similar griddle, include the cut mushrooms, cut bell pepper, snow peas, and broccoli florets. Stir-fry for around four to five mins till the vegetables are soft-crisp.

5. Return the cooked tofu to the griddle then cook for extra minute, stirring well to blend everything. Flavour with salt and pepper as required.

6. Serve warm.

Per serving: Calories: 180kcal; Fat: 10gm; Carbs: 9g; Protein: 15g; Sugar: 4g; Sodium: 190mg; Potassium: 310mg; Phosphorus: 240mg

Baked Pork Chops with Apples

Degree of Difficulty: ★★★☆☆

Preparation time: fifteen mins

Cooking time: thirty mins

Servings: two

Ingredients:

- two boneless pork chops
- one tbsp olive oil
- one tsp dried sage
- half tsp dried thyme
- quarter tsp garlic powder
- Salt and pepper as required
- one apple, skinned and cut
- half onion, thinly cut
- quarter teacup low-sodium chicken broth

Directions:

1. Warm up the oven to 375°F.
2. Flavour the pork chops with dried sage, dried thyme, garlic powder, salt, and pepper.
3. Warm your olive oil in an ovenproof griddle in a medium-high temp. Include the seasoned pork chops and cook for around three to four mins on all sides till browned.
4. Take out the griddle from the heat. Place the cut apple and thinly cut onion around the pork chops in the griddle.
5. Pour the low-sodium chicken broth into the griddle.
6. Transfer the griddle to the warmed up oven then bake for twenty to twenty-five mins or

'til the pork chops are cooked through then the apples are soft.

7. Serve warm.

Per serving: Calories: 280kcal; Fat: 12g; Carbs: 15g; Protein: 27g; Sugar: 9g; Sodium: 120mg; Potassium: 380mg; Phosphorus: 320mg

Baked Eggplant Parmesan

Degree of Difficulty: ★★★☆☆

Preparation time: thirty mins

Cooking time: thirty mins

Servings: four

Ingredients:

- one large eggplant, cut into quarter-inch rounds
- one teacup low-sodium marinara sauce
- half teacup shredded mozzarella cheese
- quarter teacup grated Parmesan cheese
- quarter teacup breadcrumbs
- half tsp dried oregano
- half tsp dried basil
- Salt and pepper as required

Directions:

1. Warm up the oven to 400°F.
2. Bring the eggplant slices on a baking tray lined with parchment paper. Spray salt on both sides of the eggplant slices then let them sit for around fifteen mins to release excess moisture. Pat dry with a paper towel.

3. Inside a small container, blend the breadcrumbs, dried oregano, dried basil, salt, and pepper.

4. Dip each eggplant slice into the breadcrumb solution, covering all ends. Put them back on the baking tray.

5. Bake the eggplant slices for fifteen-twenty mins or till golden brown and crispy.

6. In your baking tray, disperse a thin layer of marinara sauce. Arrange half of the baked eggplant slices on top. Disperse another layer of marinara sauce then spray half of the shredded mozzarella cheese and grated Parmesan cheese on top.

7. Repeat the layering process using the remaining eggplant slices, marinara sauce, and cheeses.

8. Bake for an extra fifteen mins or till the cheese is dissolved and bubbly.

9. Serve warm.

Per serving: Calories: 200kcal; Fat: 8g; Carbs: 18g; Protein: 12g; Sugar: 6g; Sodium: 320mg; Potassium: 320mg; Phosphorus: 220mg

Chicken and Mushroom Stir-Fry

Degree of Difficulty: ★★☆☆☆
Preparation time: fifteen mins
Cooking time: fifteen mins
Servings: 4
Ingredients:

- two chicken breasts, cut into strips
- one tbsp olive oil
- two pieces of garlic, crushed
- one tsp ginger, grated
- two teacups cut mushrooms
- one bell pepper, cut
- one teacup snow peas
- two tbsps low-sodium soy sauce
- one tbsp rice vinegar
- half tsp sesame oil

Directions:

1. Warm the olive oil in a huge griddle or wok at medium-high temp.

2. Include the cut chicken breasts then cook for around 5-6 mins till browned and cooked through. Take the chicken from the griddle and put away.

3. Inside your similar griddle, include the crushed garlic, grated ginger, cut mushrooms, cut bell pepper, and snow peas. Stir-fry for around four to five mins till the vegetables are soft-crisp.

4. Inside a small container, whisk collectively the low-sodium soy sauce, rice vinegar, and sesame oil.

5. Return the cooked chicken to the griddle then pour the sauce over the chicken & vegetables. Cook for another min, stirring well to cover all.

6. Serve warm.

Per serving: Calories: 200kcal; Fat: 7g; Carbs: 8g; Protein: 25g; Sugar: 3gm; Sodium: 260mg; Potassium: 240mg; Phosphorus: 200mg

Quinoa Stuffed Peppers

Degree of Difficulty: ★★★☆☆

Preparation time: twenty mins

Cooking time: forty-five mins

Servings: four

Ingredients:

- 4 bell peppers (any color), tops removed and seeds removed
- one teacup cooked quinoa
- half lb. ground turkey or chicken
- 1/2 onion, cubed
- 1 carrot, grated
- 1/2 zucchini, grated
- quarter teacup low-sodium chicken broth
- one tsp dried basil
- half tsp dried oregano
- Salt and pepper as required

Directions:

1. Warm up the oven to 375°F.
2. Blanch the bell peppers your boiling water for five mins. Take out them from the water and put away.
3. Inside a griddle, cook the ground turkey or chicken across middling temp. till browned. Include the cubed onion, grated carrot, and grated zucchini. Cook till the vegetables are soft.
4. Stir in the cooked quinoa, low-sodium chicken broth, dried basil, dried oregano, salt, and pepper. Cook for an additional two-three mins 'til warmed over.
5. Stuff the bell peppers with the quinoa and turkey or chicken solution and place them in a baking tray.
6. Bake for thirty to thirty-five mins or 'til the peppers are soft and the filling is hot.
7. Serve warm.

Per serving: Calories: 220kcal; Fat: 8g; Carbs: 24gm; Protein: 16g; Sugar: 6g; Sodium: 170mg; Potassium: 270mg; Phosphorus: 200mg

Baked Salmon with Herbed Yogurt Sauce

Degree of Difficulty: ★★☆☆☆

Preparation time: ten mins

Cooking time: twenty mins

Servings: 2

Ingredients:

- two salmon fillets
- one tbsp olive oil
- one tbsp fresh dill, severed
- one tbsp fresh parsley, severed
- one piece of garlic, crushed
- quarter teacup plain yogurt
- one tsp lemon juice

- Salt and pepper as required

Directions:

1. Warm up the oven to 400°F.

2. Bring the salmon fillets on a baking tray lined with parchment paper. Spray with olive oil then spray with fresh dill, fresh parsley, crushed garlic, salt, and pepper.

3. Bake for fifteen-twenty mins or 'til the salmon flakes simply with a fork.

4. Inside your small container, blend collectively the plain yogurt, lemon juice, salt, and pepper.

5. Serve the baked salmon with the herbed yogurt sauce on top.

Per serving: Calories: 300kcal; Fat: 18gm; Carbs: 4g; Protein: 30g; Sugar: 1g; Sodium: 100mg; Potassium: 320mg; Phosphorus: 240mg

Tuna and White Bean Salad

Degree of Difficulty: ★★☆☆☆
Preparation time: fifteen mins
Cooking time: N/A
Servings: two
Ingredients:

- one tin tuna, drained
- one tin white beans, drained and washed
- half red onion, finely severed
- quarter teacup severed fresh parsley
- one tbsp lemon juice
- one tbsp olive oil

- Salt and pepper as required

Directions:

1. Inside a container, blend the drained tuna, white beans, finely severed red onion, severed fresh parsley, lemon juice, olive oil, salt, and pepper. Toss well to blend.

2. Serve cooled.

Per serving: Calories: 280kcal; Fat: 8g; Carbs: 28g; Protein: 25g; Sugar: 1gm; Sodium: 180mg; Potassium: 370mg; Phosphorus: 200mg

Chicken and Vegetable Stir-Fry

Degree of Difficulty: ★★☆☆☆
Preparation time: fifteen mins
Cooking time: fifteen mins
Servings: 4
Ingredients:

- two chicken breasts, cut into strips
- one tbsp olive oil
- two pieces of garlic, crushed
- one tsp ginger, grated
- one teacup cut mushrooms
- one bell pepper, cut
- one teacup snow peas
- two tbsps low-sodium soy sauce
- one tbsp rice vinegar
- half tsp sesame oil

Directions:

1. Warm the olive oil in a huge griddle or wok at medium-high temp.

2. Place the cut chicken breasts and cook for around 5-6 mins till browned and cooked through. Take the chicken from the griddle and put away.

3. In your same griddle, include the crushed garlic, grated ginger, cut mushrooms, cut bell pepper, and snow peas. Stir-fry for around four to five mins till the vegetables are soft-crisp.

4. Inside a small container, whisk collectively the low-sodium soy sauce, rice vinegar, and sesame oil.

5. Return the cooked chicken to the griddle then pour the sauce across the chicken & vegetables. Cook for another min, stirring well to cover all.

6. Serve warm.

Per serving: Calories: 200kcal; Fat: 7g; Carbs: 8g; Protein: 25g; Sugar: 3gm; Sodium: 260mg; Potassium: 340mg; Phosphorus: 200mg

Greek Lemon Chicken Skewers

Degree of Difficulty: ★★☆☆☆

Preparation time: fifteen mins

Cooking time: fifteen mins

Servings: four

Ingredients:

- quarter teacup olive oil
- two tbsps lemon juice
- one tsp dried oregano
- one tsp dried thyme
- two pieces garlic, crushed
- one lb. chicken breast, that is cut into 1" cubes
- Salt and pepper as required
- half red onion, cut into wedges
- one bell pepper, cut into 1-inch pieces
- 8 cherry tomatoes
- quarter teacup crumbled feta cheese

Directions:

1. Inside your container, whisk collectively the olive oil, lemon juice, dried oregano, dried thyme, crushed garlic, salt, and pepper.

2. Bring the chicken cubes to the container and throw to cover uniformly. Marinate in the fridge for thirty mins.

3. Warm up the grill or broiler.

4. Thread the marinated chicken cubes, red onion wedges, bell pepper pieces, and cherry tomatoes onto skewers.

5. Grill or broil the skewers for around 10-fifteen mins, flipping irregularly, 'til the chicken is cooked through.

6. Spray the skewers with crumbled feta cheese prior to serving.

Per serving: Calories: 250kcal; Fat: 12g; Carbs: 7g; Protein: 29g; Sugar: 3g; Sodium: 180mg; Potassium: 340mg; Phosphorus: 200

Salad Recipes

Watermelon and Feta Salad

Degree of Difficulty: ★☆☆☆☆

Preparation time: ten mins

Cooking time: zero mins

Servings: two

Ingredients:

- two teacups cubed watermelon
- quarter teacup crumbled feta cheese
- two tbsps severed fresh mint leaves
- one tbsp balsamic vinegar
- one tsp olive oil

Directions:

1. Inside a big container, blend the watermelon, feta cheese, and mint leaves.
2. Inside your small container, whisk collectively the balsamic vinegar and olive oil.
3. Transfer the dressing across the salad and throw gently to blend.
4. Serve cooled.

Per serving: Calories: 120kcal; Fat: 6gm; Carbs: 12g; Protein: 4g; Sugar: 10g; Sodium: 160mg; Potassium: 320mg; Phosphorus: 120mg

Broccoli and Cranberry Salad

Degree of Difficulty: ★★☆☆☆

Preparation time: fifteen mins

Cooking time: zero mins

Servings: two

Ingredients:

- two teacups severed broccoli florets
- quarter teacup dried cranberries
- two tbsps severed red onion
- two tbsps severed almonds
- one tbsp apple cider vinegar
- one tbsp olive oil
- one tsp honey

Directions:

1. Inside a big container, blend the broccoli florets, dried cranberries, red onion, and almonds.
2. Inside your small container, whisk collectively the apple cider vinegar, olive oil, and honey.
3. Transfer the dressing across the salad and throw well to cover.
4. Serve cooled.

Per serving: Calories: 160kcal; Fat: 9g; Carbs: 18gm; Protein: 4gm; Sugar: 9g; Sodium: 40mg; Potassium: 330mg; Phosphorus: 80mg

Spinach and Strawberry Salad

Degree of Difficulty: ★★☆☆☆

Preparation time: fifteen mins

Cooking time: zero mins

Servings: 2

Ingredients:

- two teacups fresh spinach leaves
- one teacup cut strawberries
- quarter teacup crumbled feta cheese
- two tbsps severed almonds
- one tbsp balsamic vinegar
- one tsp honey

Directions:

1. Inside a big container, blend the spinach, strawberries, feta cheese, and almonds.
2. Inside your small container, whisk collectively the balsamic vinegar and honey.
3. Transfer the dressing across the salad and throw gently to cover.
4. Serve instantly.

Per serving: Calories: 150kcal; Fat: 9gm; Carbs: 14g; Protein: 5g; Sugar: 8g; Sodium: 170mg; Potassium: 370mg; Phosphorus: 100mg

Cucumber and Tomato Salad

Degree of Difficulty: ★☆☆☆☆

Preparation time: ten mins

Cooking time: zero mins

Servings: 2

Ingredients:

- 1 cucumber, cut
- 2 tomatoes, cubed
- quarter red onion, thinly cut
- two tbsps severed fresh parsley
- one tbsp olive oil
- one tbsp lemon juice
- Salt and pepper as required

Directions:

1. Inside your container, blend the cucumber, tomatoes, red onion, and parsley.
2. Inside a distinct small container, whisk collectively the olive oil, lemon juice, salt, and pepper.
3. Transfer the dressing across the salad and throw to blend.
4. Serve cooled.

Per serving: Calories: 90kcal; Fat: 6gm; Carbs: 8gm; Protein: 2gm; Sugar: 4g; Sodium: 10mg; Potassium: 280mg; Phosphorus: 40mg

Lentil and Vegetable Salad

Degree of Difficulty: ★★☆☆☆

Preparation time: fifteen mins

Cooking time: twenty mins

Servings: 2

Ingredients:

- one teacup cooked lentils
- half teacup cubed bell peppers

- half teacup cubed zucchini
- quarter teacup severed red onion
- two tbsps severed fresh cilantro
- one tbsp lemon juice
- one tbsp olive oil
- Salt and pepper as required

Directions:

1. Inside a big container, blend the cooked lentils, cubed bell peppers, cubed zucchini, red onion, and cilantro.

2. Inside your small container, whisk collectively the lemon juice, olive oil, salt, and pepper.

3. Transfer the dressing across the salad and throw well to blend.

4. Serve cooled.

Per serving: Calories: 230kcal; Fat: 7gm; Carbs: 32g; Protein: 12gm; Sugar: 6g; Sodium: 15mg; Potassium: 360mg; Phosphorus: 190mg

Radish and Snap Pea Salad

Degree of Difficulty: ★☆☆☆☆

Preparation time: fifteen mins

Cooking time: zero mins

Servings: two

Ingredients:

- one teacup cut radishes
- one teacup snap peas, cut diagonally
- two tbsps severed fresh mint leaves
- one tbsp rice vinegar

- one tbsp sesame oil
- Salt and pepper as required

Directions:

1. Inside a big container, blend the cut radishes, snap peas, and severed mint leaves.

2. Inside your small container, whisk collectively the rice vinegar, sesame oil, salt, and pepper.

3. Transfer the dressing across the salad and throw gently to blend.

4. Serve cooled.

Per serving: Calories: 60kcal; Fat: 4g; Carbs: 6gm; Protein: 2gm; Sugar: 2gm; Sodium: 10mg; Potassium: 180mg; Phosphorus: 40mg

Egg and Asparagus Salad

Degree of Difficulty: ★★★★☆

Preparation time: twenty mins

Cooking time: ten mins

Servings: two

Ingredients:

- four hard-boiled eggs, cut
- one teacup cooked asparagus, cut into pieces
- two teacups mixed salad greens
- two tbsps cut almonds
- one tbsp lemon juice
- one tbsp olive oil
- Salt and pepper as required

Directions:

1. Inside a big container, blend the cut hard-boiled eggs, cooked asparagus, and mixed salad greens.
2. Inside your small container, whisk collectively the lemon juice, olive oil, salt, and pepper.
3. Transfer the dressing across the salad and throw gently to blend.
4. Spray cut almonds on top.
5. Serve cooled.

Per serving: Calories: 230kcal; Fat: 17g; Carbs: 9g; Protein: 12g; Sugar: 3g; Sodium: 140mg; Potassium: 320mg; Phosphorus: 200mg

Beet and Orange Salad

Degree of Difficulty: ★★☆☆☆

Preparation time: fifteen mins

Cooking time: zero mins

Servings: two

Ingredients:

- 2 medium beets, cooked and cubed
- two oranges, skinned and segmented
- two teacups mixed salad greens
- two tbsps crumbled goat cheese
- one tbsp balsamic vinegar
- one tbsp olive oil
- Salt and pepper as required

Directions:

1. Inside a big bowl, blend the cubed beets, orange segments, and mixed salad greens.
2. Inside your small container, whisk collectively the balsamic vinegar, olive oil, salt, and pepper.
3. Transfer the dressing across the salad and throw gently to blend.
4. Spray crumbled goat cheese on top.
5. Serve cooled.

Per serving: Calories: 170kcal; Fat: 7g; Carbs: 25g; Protein: 4g; Sugar: 17g; Sodium: 130mg; Potassium: 300mg; Phosphorus: 110mg

Chicken and Apple Salad

Degree of Difficulty: ★★☆☆☆

Preparation time: twenty mins

Cooking time: fifteen mins

Servings: 2

Ingredients:

- one cooked chicken breast, shredded
- one apple, cubed
- quarter teacup severed celery
- two tbsps severed walnuts
- two tbsps plain yogurt
- one tbsp lemon juice
- one tbsp severed fresh dill
- Salt and pepper as required

Directions:

1. Inside a big container, blend the shredded chicken, cubed apple, celery, and walnuts.

2. Inside your small container, blend collectively the plain yogurt, salt, lemon juice, severed fresh dill and pepper.

3. Transfer the dressing across the salad and throw gently to cover.

4. Serve cooled.

Per serving: Calories: 230kcal; Fat: 12g; Carbs: 13g; Protein: 20g; Sugar: 8g; Sodium: 80mg; Potassium: 370mg; Phosphorus: 200mg

Avocado and Shrimp Salad

Degree of Difficulty: ★★★☆☆

Preparation time: twenty mins

Cooking time: five mins

Servings: 2

Ingredients:

- half lb. cooked shrimp, skinned & deveined
- 1 avocado, cubed
- quarter teacup cubed red bell pepper
- two tbsps severed cilantro
- one tbsp lime juice
- one tbsp olive oil
- Salt and pepper as required

Directions:

1. Inside a big container, blend the shrimp, avocado, red bell pepper, and cilantro.

2. Inside your small container, whisk collectively the lime juice, olive oil, salt, and pepper.

3. Transfer the dressing across the salad and throw gently to blend.

4. Serve cooled.

Per serving: Calories: 250kcal; Fat: 16g; Carbs: 8gm; Protein: 20g; Sugar: 1gm; Sodium: 200mg; Potassium: 310mg; Phosphorus: 200mg

Roasted Brussels Sprouts Salad

Degree of Difficulty: ★★★★☆

Preparation time: fifteen mins

Cooking time: twenty-five mins

Servings: 2

Ingredients:

- two teacups roasted Brussels sprouts, halved
- quarter teacup severed walnuts
- two tbsps dried cranberries
- one tbsp balsamic vinegar
- one tbsp olive oil
- Salt and pepper as required

Directions:

1. Inside a big container, blend the roasted Brussels sprouts, severed walnuts, and dried cranberries.

2. Inside your small container, whisk collectively the balsamic vinegar, olive oil, salt, and pepper.

3. Transfer the dressing across the salad and throw gently to blend.

4. Serve cooled.

Per serving: Calories: 220kcal; Fat: 17gm; Carbs: 17g; Protein: 6gm; Sugar: 7g; Sodium: 40mg; Potassium: 360mg; Phosphorus: 110mg

Turkey and Cranberry Salad

Degree of Difficulty: ★★☆☆☆

Preparation time: fifteen mins

Cooking time: ten mins

Servings: two

Ingredients:

- 4 ounces cooked turkey breast, shredded
- quarter teacup dried cranberries
- two tbsps severed pecans
- two tbsps plain yogurt
- one tbsp mayonnaise
- one tsp Dijon mustard
- Salt and pepper as required

Directions:

1. Inside a big container, blend the shredded turkey breast, dried cranberries, and severed pecans.
2. Inside your small container, blend collectively the plain yogurt, mayonnaise, Dijon mustard, salt, and pepper.
3. Transfer the dressing across the salad and throw gently to cover.
4. Serve cooled.

Per serving: Calories: 260kcal; Fat: 13g; Carbs: 17g; Protein: 19g; Sugar: 10g; Sodium: 130mg; Potassium: 280mg; Phosphorus: 230mg

Shrimp and Mango Salad

Degree of Difficulty: ★★★☆☆

Preparation time: twenty mins

Cooking time: five mins

Servings: 2

Ingredients:

- half lb. cooked shrimp, skinned & deveined
- 1 ripe mango, cubed
- quarter teacup cubed red onion
- two tbsps severed fresh cilantro
- one tbsp lime juice
- one tbsp olive oil
- Salt and pepper as required

Directions:

1. Inside a big container, blend the cooked shrimp, cubed mango, red onion, and cilantro.
2. Inside your small container, whisk collectively the lime juice, olive oil, salt, and pepper.
3. Transfer the dressing across the salad and throw gently to blend.
4. Serve cooled.

Per serving: Calories: 220kcal; Fat: 7gm; Carbs: 21g; Protein: 19gm; Sugar: 16g; Sodium: 230mg; Potassium: 380mg; Phosphorus: 200mg

Arugula and Pomegranate Salad

Degree of Difficulty: ★☆☆☆☆

Preparation time: ten mins

Cooking time: zero mins

Servings: 2

Ingredients:

- two teacups arugula
- half teacup pomegranate seeds
- two tbsps crumbled goat cheese
- one tbsp balsamic vinegar
- one tbsp olive oil
- one tsp honey

Directions:

1. Inside a big container, blend the arugula, pomegranate seeds, and crumbled goat cheese.

2. Inside your small container, whisk collectively the balsamic vinegar, olive oil, and honey.

3. Transfer the dressing across the salad and throw gently to blend.

4. Serve cooled.

Per serving: Calories: 120kcal; Fat: 7gm; Carbs: 10g; Protein: 3g; Sugar: 7gm; Sodium: 90mg; Potassium: 240mg; Phosphorus: 80mg

Kale and Quinoa Salad

Degree of Difficulty: ★★☆☆☆

Preparation time: twenty mins

Cooking time: fifteen mins

Servings: 2

Ingredients:

- two teacups severed kale leaves
- one teacup cooked quinoa
- quarter teacup cubed cucumber
- two tbsps severed roasted almonds
- one tbsp lemon juice
- one tbsp olive oil
- Salt and pepper as required

Directions:

1. Inside a big container, blend the severed kale leaves, cooked quinoa, cubed cucumber, and severed roasted almonds.

2. Inside your small container, whisk collectively the lemon juice, olive oil, salt, and pepper.

3. Transfer the dressing across the salad and throw well to cover.

4. Serve cooled.

Per serving: Calories: 250kcal; Fat: 13g; Carbs: 26g; Protein: 9gm; Sugar: 2gm; Sodium: 30mg; Potassium: 360mg; Phosphorus: 180mg

Mushroom and Arugula Salad

Degree of Difficulty: ★★☆☆☆

Preparation time: fifteen mins

Cooking time: ten mins

Servings: two

Ingredients:

- two teacups cut mushrooms
- two teacups arugula
- two tbsps cut almonds
- one tbsp balsamic vinegar
- one tbsp olive oil
- Salt and pepper as required

Directions:

1. Inside a big griddle, sauté the cut mushrooms in olive oil till soft.
2. Inside a big container, blend the sautéed mushrooms, arugula, and cut almonds.
3. Inside your small container, whisk collectively the balsamic vinegar, olive oil, salt, and pepper.
4. Transfer the dressing across the salad and throw gently to blend.
5. Serve cooled.

Per serving: Calories: 130kcal; Fat: 10gm; Carbs: 8g; Protein: 5gm; Sugar: 3g; Sodium: 10mg; Potassium: 370mg; Phosphorus: 120mg

Apple and Walnut Salad

Degree of Difficulty: ★☆☆☆☆

Preparation time: ten mins

Cooking time: zero mins

Servings: 2

Ingredients:

- two teacups mixed salad greens
- one apple, thinly cut
- quarter teacup severed walnuts
- two tbsps crumbled blue cheese
- one tbsp apple cider vinegar
- one tbsp olive oil
- Salt and pepper as required

Directions:

1. Inside a big container, blend the mixed salad greens, apple slices, severed walnuts, and crumbled blue cheese.
2. Inside your small container, whisk collectively the apple cider vinegar, olive oil, salt, and pepper.
3. Transfer the dressing across the salad and throw gently to blend.
4. Serve cooled.

Per serving: Calories: 200kcal; Fat: 16g; Carbs: 12g; Protein: 4g; Sugar: 7g; Sodium: 200mg; Potassium: 220mg; Phosphorus: 80mg

Caprese Salad

Degree of Difficulty: ★☆☆☆☆

Preparation time: ten mins

Cooking time: zero mins

Servings: two

Ingredients:

- 2 medium tomatoes, cut
- 4 ounces fresh mozzarella cheese, cut
- quarter teacup fresh basil leaves
- one tbsp balsamic vinegar
- one tbsp olive oil
- Salt and pepper as required

Directions:

1. On a serving plate, alternate slices of tomatoes and fresh mozzarella cheese.

2. Tuck fresh basil leaves in between the tomato and cheese slices.

3. Inside your small container, whisk collectively the balsamic vinegar, olive oil, salt, and pepper.

4. Spray the dressing across the salad.

5. Serve cooled.

Per serving: Calories: 200kcal; Fat: 16gm; Carbs: 6g; Protein: 12g; Sugar: 4g; Sodium: 240mg; Potassium: 350mg; Phosphorus: 220mg

Radicchio and Orange Salad

Degree of Difficulty: ★★☆☆☆

Preparation time: fifteen mins

Cooking time: zero mins

Servings: 2

Ingredients:

- two teacups shredded radicchio
- two oranges, skinned and segmented
- two tbsps severed toasted walnuts
- one tbsp balsamic vinegar
- one tbsp olive oil
- Salt and pepper as required

Directions:

1. Inside a big container, blend the shredded radicchio, orange segments, and severed toasted walnuts.

2. Inside your small container, whisk collectively the balsamic vinegar, olive oil, salt, and pepper.

3. Transfer the dressing across the salad and throw gently to blend.

4. Serve cooled.

Per serving: Calories: 180kcal; Fat: 12gm; Carbs: 18g; Protein: 3gm; Sugar: 12g; Sodium: 10mg; Potassium: 350mg; Phosphorus: 70mg

Chickpea and Tomato Salad

Degree of Difficulty: ★★☆☆☆

Preparation time: fifteen mins

Cooking time: zero mins

Servings: two

Ingredients:

- one tin chickpeas, rinsed and drained
- one teacup cubed tomatoes
- quarter teacup cubed cucumber
- two tbsps severed fresh parsley
- one tbsp lemon juice
- one tbsp olive oil
- Salt and pepper as required

Directions:

1. Inside a big container, blend the chickpeas, cubed tomatoes, cubed cucumber, and parsley.

2. Inside your small container, whisk collectively the lemon juice, olive oil, salt, and pepper.

3. Transfer the dressing across the salad and throw well to cover.

4. Serve cooled.

Per serving: Calories: 240kcal; Fat: 8g; Carbs: 35g; Protein: 11g; Sugar: 7g; Sodium: 240mg; Potassium: 380mg; Phosphorus: 190mg

Conversion Chart

Volume Equivalents (Liquid)

US Standard	US Standard (ounces)	Metric (approximate)
two tbsps	1 fl. oz.	30 milliliter
quarter teacup	2 fl. oz.	60 milliliter
half teacup	4 fl. oz.	120 milliliter
one teacup	8 fl. oz.	240 milliliter
one and half teacups	12 fl. oz.	355 milliliter
two teacups or one pint	16 fl. oz.	475 milliliter
four teacups or one quart	32 fl. oz.	1 Liter
one gallon	128 fl. oz.	4 Liter

Volume Equivalents (Dry)

US Standard	Metric (approximate)
one-eighth tsp	0.5 milliliter
quarter tsp	1 milliliter
half tsp	2 milliliter
three-quarter tsp	4 milliliter
one tsp	5 milliliter
one tbsp	15 milliliter
quarter teacup	59 milliliter
one-third teacup	79 milliliter
half teacup	118 milliliter
two-third teacup	156 milliliter
three-quarter teacup	177 milliliter
one teacup	235 milliliter
two teacups or one pint	475 milliliter
three teacups	700 milliliter

four teacups or one quart	1 Liter

Oven Temperatures

Fahrenheit (F)	Celsius (C) (approximate)
250 deg. F	120 deg. C
300 deg. F	150 deg. C
325 deg. F	165 deg. C
350 deg. F	180 deg. C
375 deg. F	190 deg. C
400 deg. F	200 deg. C
425 deg. F	220 deg. C
450 deg. F	230 deg. C

Weight Equivalents

US Standard	Metric (approximate)
one tbsp	15 gm
half oz.	15 gm
one oz.	30 gm
two oz.	60 gm
four oz.	115 gm
eight oz.	225 gm
twelve oz.	340 gm
sixteen oz. or one lb.	455 gm

8 - Weeks Meal Plan

Week 1:

Day	Breakfast	Lunch	Dinner	Dessert
1	Vegetable Frittata	Quinoa and Vegetable Stir-Fry	Lemon Garlic Roasted Chicken Thighs	Pears with Honey and Cinnamon
2	Greek Yogurt with Honey and Nuts	Lentil and Vegetable Curry	Grilled Balsamic Pork Chops	Coconut Rice Pudding
3	Blueberry Chia Pudding	Tofu Stir-Fry with Vegetables	Grilled Lemon Herb Tofu	Chocolate Mousse
4	Sweet Potato Hash Browns	Greek Salad with Grilled Chicken	Baked Lemon Dill Salmon	Lemon Yogurt Cake
5	Veggie Breakfast Burrito	Cauliflower Rice Stir-Fry with Chicken	Beef and Vegetable Stir-Fry	Watermelon Granita
6	Cottage Cheese with Fresh Fruit	Spinach and Mushroom Stuffed Chicken Breast	Quinoa and Vegetable Stuffed Bell Peppers	Strawberry Frozen Yogurt
7	Scrambled Eggs with Vegetables	Grilled Shrimp Skewers with Lemon Garlic Sauce	Baked Cod with Roasted Vegetables	Baked Peaches with Cinnamon

Week 2:

Day	Breakfast	Lunch	Dinner	Dessert
1	Whole Wheat Toast with Avocado	Grilled Vegetable Skewers	Grilled Chicken and Vegetable Skewers	Lemon Poppy Seed Muffins
2	Yogurt Parfait	Quinoa Breakfast Bowl	Baked Cod with Lemon Caper Sauce	Pineapple Coconut Smoothie

3	Greek Yogurt with Honey and Nuts	Grilled Lemon Herb Tofu	Beef Kabobs with Pepper	Baked Apples with Cinnamon
4	Veggie Breakfast Burrito	Tuna Salad Lettuce Wraps	Roasted Salmon with Dill	Vanilla Rice Pudding
5	Egg and Vegetable Muffins	Greek-Style Roasted Vegetables	Baked Lemon Herb Chicken	Mango Yogurt Parfait
6	Oatmeal with Fresh Berries	Baked Pork Chops with Rosemary	Turkey Meatballs with Marinara Sauce	Honeydew Lime Sorbet
7	Vegetable Frittata	Spinach and Mushroom Omelet	Baked Chicken and Vegetable Casserole	Blueberry Oat Bars

Week 3:

Day	Breakfast	Lunch	Dinner	Dessert
1	Cinnamon Apple Pancakes	Shrimp Stir-Fry	Baked Cod with Roasted Vegetables	Lemon Yogurt Cake
2	Fruit Salad with Mint	Caprese Salad with Grilled Chicken	Quinoa and Vegetable Stuffed Bell Peppers	Watermelon Granita
3	Blueberry Chia Pudding	Vegetarian Gobi Curry	Grilled Lemon Herb Tofu	Coconut Rice Pudding
4	Easy Turnip Puree	Grilled Shrimp Skewers with Lemon Garlic Sauce	Grilled Balsamic Pork Chops	Pineapple Coconut Smoothie
5	Egg and Vegetable Muffins	Quinoa and Black Bean Salad	Baked Lemon Dill Salmon	Strawberry Frozen Yogurt
6	Spinach and Feta Egg Muffins	Grilled Vegetable Skewers	Grilled Chicken and Vegetable Skewers	Apple Cinnamon Muffins

7	Greek Yogurt with Honey and Nuts	Lentil and Vegetable Curry	Lemon Garlic Roasted Chicken Thighs	Baked Apples with Cinnamon

Week 4:

Day	Breakfast	Lunch	Dinner	Dessert
1	Whole Wheat Toast with Avocado	Spinach and Mushroom Stuffed Chicken Breast	Beef and Vegetable Stir-Fry	Lemon Poppy Seed Muffins
2	Yogurt Parfait	Quinoa Breakfast Bowl	Baked Cod with Lemon Caper Sauce	Pineapple Coconut Smoothie
3	Greek Yogurt with Honey and Nuts	Tofu Stir-Fry with Vegetables	Beef Kabobs with Pepper	Baked Apples with Cinnamon
4	Veggie Breakfast Burrito	Greek-Style Roasted Vegetables	Baked Lemon Herb Chicken	Mango Yogurt Parfait
5	Egg and Vegetable Muffins	Shrimp and Asparagus Stir-Fry	Turkey Meatballs with Marinara Sauce	Honeydew Lime Sorbet
6	Oatmeal with Fresh Berries	Baked Pork Chops with Rosemary	Baked Chicken and Vegetable Casserole	Blueberry Oat Bars
7	Vegetable Frittata	Grilled Turkey Burgers	Grilled Salmon with Herbed Quinoa	Watermelon Granita

Week 5:

Day	Breakfast	Lunch	Dinner	Dessert
1	Sweet Potato Hash Browns	Quinoa and Vegetable Stir-Fry	Lemon Garlic Roasted Chicken Thighs	Pears with Honey and Cinnamon
2	Greek Yogurt with Honey and Nuts	Lentil and Vegetable Curry	Grilled Balsamic Pork Chops	Coconut Rice Pudding

3	Blueberry Chia Pudding	Tofu Stir-Fry with Vegetables	Grilled Lemon Herb Tofu	Chocolate Mousse
4	Fruit Salad with Mint	Greek Salad with Grilled Chicken	Baked Lemon Dill Salmon	Lemon Yogurt Cake
5	Veggie Breakfast Burrito	Cauliflower Rice Stir-Fry with Chicken	Beef and Vegetable Stir-Fry	Watermelon Granita
6	Cottage Cheese with Fresh Fruit	Spinach and Mushroom Stuffed Chicken Breast	Quinoa and Vegetable Stuffed Bell Peppers	Strawberry Frozen Yogurt
7	Scrambled Eggs with Vegetables	Grilled Shrimp Skewers with Lemon Garlic Sauce	Baked Cod with Roasted Vegetables	Baked Peaches with Cinnamon

Week 6:

Day	Breakfast	Lunch	Dinner	Dessert
1	Cinnamon Apple Pancakes	Shrimp Stir-Fry	Baked Cod with Roasted Vegetables	Lemon Yogurt Cake
2	Fruit Salad with Mint	Caprese Salad with Grilled Chicken	Quinoa and Vegetable Stuffed Bell Peppers	Watermelon Granita
3	Blueberry Chia Pudding	Vegetarian Gobi Curry	Grilled Lemon Herb Tofu	Coconut Rice Pudding
4	Easy Turnip Puree	Grilled Shrimp Skewers with Lemon Garlic Sauce	Grilled Balsamic Pork Chops	Pineapple Coconut Smoothie
5	Egg and Vegetable Muffins	Quinoa and Black Bean Salad	Baked Lemon Dill Salmon	Strawberry Frozen Yogurt
6	Spinach and Feta Egg Muffins	Grilled Vegetable Skewers	Grilled Chicken and Vegetable Skewers	Apple Cinnamon Muffins

7	Greek Yogurt with Honey and Nuts	Lentil and Vegetable Curry	Lemon Garlic Roasted Chicken Thighs	Baked Apples with Cinnamon

Week 7:

Day	Breakfast	Lunch	Dinner	Dessert
1	Whole Wheat Toast with Avocado	Spinach and Mushroom Stuffed Chicken Breast	Beef and Vegetable Stir-Fry	Lemon Poppy Seed Muffins
2	Yogurt Parfait	Quinoa Breakfast Bowl	Baked Cod with Lemon Caper Sauce	Pineapple Coconut Smoothie
3	Greek Yogurt with Honey and Nuts	Tofu Stir-Fry with Vegetables	Beef Kabobs with Pepper	Baked Apples with Cinnamon
4	Veggie Breakfast Burrito	Greek-Style Roasted Vegetables	Baked Lemon Herb Chicken	Mango Yogurt Parfait
5	Egg and Vegetable Muffins	Shrimp and Asparagus Stir-Fry	Turkey Meatballs with Marinara Sauce	Honeydew Lime Sorbet
6	Oatmeal with Fresh Berries	Baked Pork Chops with Rosemary	Baked Chicken and Vegetable Casserole	Blueberry Oat Bars
7	Vegetable Frittata	Grilled Turkey Burgers	Grilled Salmon with Herbed Quinoa	Watermelon Granita

Week 8:

Day	Breakfast	Lunch	Dinner	Dessert
1	Sweet Potato Hash Browns	Quinoa and Vegetable Stir-Fry	Lemon Garlic Roasted Chicken Thighs	Pears with Honey and Cinnamon

2	Greek Yogurt with Honey and Nuts	Lentil and Vegetable Curry	Grilled Balsamic Pork Chops	Coconut Rice Pudding
3	Blueberry Chia Pudding	Tofu Stir-Fry with Vegetables	Grilled Lemon Herb Tofu	Chocolate Mousse
4	Fruit Salad with Mint	Greek Salad with Grilled Chicken	Baked Lemon Dill Salmon	Lemon Yogurt Cake
5	Veggie Breakfast Burrito	Cauliflower Rice Stir-Fry with Chicken	Beef and Vegetable Stir-Fry	Watermelon Granita
6	Cottage Cheese with Fresh Fruit	Spinach and Mushroom Stuffed Chicken Breast	Quinoa and Vegetable Stuffed Bell Peppers	Strawberry Frozen Yogurt
7	Scrambled Eggs with Vegetables	Grilled Shrimp Skewers with Lemon Garlic Sauce	Baked Cod with Roasted Vegetables	Baked Peaches with Cinnamon

Index

Grilled Salmon with Dill Sauce; 81
Grilled Salmon with Herbed Quinoa; 46
Grilled Shrimp Skewers with Lemon Garlic Sauce; 37
Grilled Turkey Burgers; 28
Grilled Vegetable Skewers; 36
Ham and Cheese Omelet; 26
Honeydew Lime Sorbet; 76
Kale and Quinoa Salad; 98
Lemon Garlic Roasted Chicken Thighs; 44
Lemon Garlic Shrimp Skewers; 53
Lemon Poppy Seed Muffins; 75
Lemon Yogurt Cake; 78
Lentil and Vegetable Curry; 33
Lentil and Vegetable Salad; 93
Mango Yogurt Parfait; 77
Melon and Prosciutto Roll-Ups; 61
Mushroom and Arugula Salad; 98
Oatmeal with Fresh Berries; 17
Orange Sherbet; 69
Peach Crumble; 76
Pears with Honey and Cinnamon; 69
Pineapple Coconut Smoothie; 71
Quinoa and Black Bean Salad; 35
Quinoa and Vegetable Salad; 85
Quinoa and Vegetable Stir-Fry; 28
Quinoa and Vegetable Stuffed Bell Peppers; 50
Quinoa Breakfast Bowl; 22
Quinoa Salad Cups; 60
Quinoa Stuffed Peppers; 89
Radicchio and Orange Salad; 100
Radish and Snap Pea Salad; 94
Raspberry Chia Jam; 71
Rice Cake with Tuna Salad; 57
Roasted Brussels Sprouts Salad; 96
Roasted Cauliflower and Chickpea Salad; 83
Roasted Chicken and Vegetables; 85
Roasted Chickpeas; 59

Roasted Herb Chicken Thighs with Steamed Vegetables; 55
Roasted Salmon with Dill; 41
Roasted Vegetable Medley; 82
Scrambled Eggs with Vegetables; 21
Shrimp and Asparagus Stir-Fry; 49
Shrimp and Broccoli Stir-Fry; 83
Shrimp and Mango Salad; 97
Shrimp Bruschetta; 20
Shrimp Stir-Fry; 29
Spinach and Feta Egg Muffins; 17
Spinach and Feta Stuffed Chicken Breast; 32
Spinach and Feta Stuffed Mushrooms; 65
Spinach and Mushroom Omelet; 52
Spinach and Mushroom Stuffed Chicken Breast; 34
Spinach and Strawberry Salad; 93
Strawberry Frozen Yogurt; 70
Stuffed Bell Peppers; 84
Sweet Potato Hash Browns; 19
Tofu Stir-Fry; 86
Tofu Stir-Fry with Vegetables; 36
Tuna and White Bean Salad; 90
Tuna Salad Lettuce Wraps; 38
Turkey and Cranberry Salad; 97
Turkey and Vegetable Skewers; 82
Turkey and Vegetable Skillet; 55
Turkey Chili; 48
Turkey Lettuce Wraps; 63
Turkey Meatballs with Marinara Sauce; 43
Vanilla Rice Pudding; 74
Vegetable and Egg Wrap; 21
Vegetable Crudité Platter; 57
Vegetable Frittata; 22
Vegetable Stir-Fry; 80
Vegetable Stir-Fry with Shrimp; 43
Vegetarian Gobi Curry; 38
Veggie Breakfast Burrito; 25

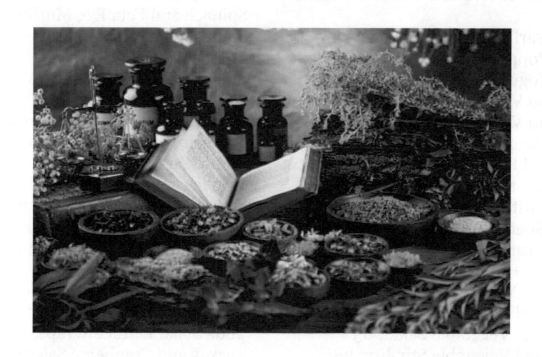

Conclusion

The renal diet is a key component of managing kidney health, especially in individuals with kidney problems like chronic kidney disease. By following the principles of the renal diet, which include limiting sodium, potassium, phosphorus, and protein intake, individuals can help preserve kidney function, control blood pressure, maintain electrolyte balance, and prevent further complications.

Adhering to a renal diet requires making thoughtful food choices and adopting healthy eating habits. It is essential to work closely with healthcare professionals, such as nephrologists and registered dietitians, who can provide personalized guidance and support in developing a suitable meal plan based on individual needs and stage of kidney disease.

While the renal diet emphasizes restrictions on certain nutrients, it is crucial to ensure adequate nutrition. This may involve selecting alternative food options, portion control, and considering the use of dietary supplements if necessary. Regular monitoring of kidney function and nutritional status is important to make any necessary adjustments to the diet plan.

In addition to dietary modifications, other lifestyle factors such as maintaining a healthy weight, staying hydrated, managing blood sugar levels (for individuals with diabetes), and avoiding tobacco & excessive alcohol consumption are also vital for overall kidney health.

By incorporating the principles of the renal diet into daily life and maintaining a holistic approach to kidney health, individuals can optimize their well-being, slow the progression of kidney disease, and improve their quality of life.